DIAGNOSTIC PROBLEMS IN BONE TUMORS: SELECTED TOPICS

DIAGNOSTIC PROBLEMS IN BONE TUMORS: SELECTED TOPICS

DIAGNOSTIC PROBLEMS IN TUMOR PATHOLOGY SERIES

Series editors

Arun Chitale, MD (Path)

Diplomate American Board of Pathology (1969)

Surgical Pathologist

Sir HN Hospital, Jaslok Hospital, Surgical Pathology Center

Formerly Professor & Head Department of Pathology Bombay Hospital Institute of Medical Sciences, Mumbai, India

Dhananjay Chitale, MD (Path) DNB (Path)

Diplomate American Board of Pathology

Vice-Chair, Anatomic Pathology

Division Head, Molecular Pathology & Genomic Medicine,

Senior Staff Surgical Pathologist

Director, Tissue Biorepository and IHC core

Assistant Clinical Professor, Wayne State University School of Medicine

Henry Ford Hospital, Detroit, Michigan, USA

Diagnostic Problems in Tumors of Head and Neck: Selected Topics, 1/e
Arun Chitale, Dhananjay Chitale, 2014

Diagnostic Problems in Tumors of Gastrointestinal tract: Selected Topics, 1/e
Arun Chitale, Dhananjay Chitale, 2014

Diagnostic Problems in Tumors of Female Genital Tract: Selected Topics, 1/e
Kedar Deodhar, Arun Chitale, 2014

Diagnostic Problems in Tumors of Central Nervous System: Selected Topics, 1/e
Arun Chitale, 2014

Diagnostic Problems in Tumors of Endocrine system: Selected Topics, 1/e
Arun Chitale, Dhananjay Chitale, 2014

Diagnostic Problems in Tumors of Bone: Selected Topics, 1/e
Ramesh Deshpande, Arun Chitale, Manish Agarwal, 2016

DIAGNOSTIC PROBLEMS IN BONE TUMORS SELECTED TOPICS

Authors

Ramesh B. Deshpande, MD (Path)

Consultant Surgical Pathologist

P.D. Hinduja National Hospital and Medical Research Centre, Mahim, Mumbai

Arun Chitale, MD (Path), DABP

Diplomate American Board of Pathology (1969)

Surgical Pathologist

Sir HN Hospital, Jaslok Hospital, Surgical Pathology Centre

Formerly Professor & Head Department of Pathology Bombay Hospital Institute of Medical Sciences, Mumbai, India

Manish Agarwal, MS (Ortho), DNB (Ortho)

Consultant Orthopedic Oncologist

P.D. Hinduja National Hospital and Medical Research Centre, Mahim, Mumbai

Honorary Orthopedic Oncologist

B J Wadia Children's Hospital, Mumbai, and T N Medical College and B Y L Nair Hospital, Mumbai, India.

Contributor:

Dhananjay A Chitale, MD, DNB, (Path) DABP

Vice-Chair, Anatomic Pathology

Division Head, Molecular Pathology & Genomic Medicine,

Senior Staff Surgical Pathologist

Director, Tissue Biorepository and IHC core

Assistant Clinical Professor, Wayne State University School of Medicine

Henry Ford Hospital, Detroit, Michigan, USA

Table of Contents

PREFACE:

DIAGNOSTIC PROBLEMS IN SURGICAL PATHOLOGY:

Uncommon presentation of common lesions and rare lesions

Histopathological evaluation is the gold standard in the diagnosis of malignant tumors and chronic diseases of visceral organs like liver, kidney and lungs. Histopathological analysis provides information that helps the clinician to choose the most appropriate treatment modality and assists in prognostication. Notwithstanding the current and future advances in the imaging technology and other innovations, the status of Histopathology will remain unchanged for decades to come.

Whereas Histopathology is the most objective form of investigation, there are many gray areas in arriving at a definitive diagnosis. On many occasions total lack of clinical information leads to avoidable errors in the diagnosis. The surgical pathologist is advised to keep the cases pending until adequate information is available. On the other hand, there are numerous problems in histological interpretation even if the entire clinical information is at hand. This occurs because some lesions have inherent morphological ambiguities and no two surgical pathologists may agree on the correct histological diagnosis. One such lesion, for example, is verrucous squamous cell carcinoma of the oro-pharyngeal region or other organs with squamous epithelial lining. The most controversial problem in thyroid disorders is a lesion called follicular variant of papillary carcinoma. In every organ and system, there are sporadic entities, which have debatable criteria of morphological diagnosis. The object of this book is to adequately address problems of uncommon morphologic variations of common lesions and rare difficult lesions with the help of extensive illustrations. There are excellent frequently updated textbooks of surgical pathology, in which all lesions occurring in various sites are described, illustrated and backed by references. However, due to constraints of space, these problematic entities are not extensively illustrated or explained at length. This deficiency is admirably handled in exclusively individual organ pathology monograms. However, this requires the facility of a well-stocked library, which may not be available in all institutions, particularly in less developed countries.

The proposed book is an attempt to address these lesions with multiple illustrations and detailed pertinent text. It is envisaged that the book should be a companion to a standard surgical pathology textbook and this should be accessible just at the fingertips via power of electronic media using internet. The targeted audience includes residents in Anatomic Pathology; young recently qualified pathologists and a large contingent of pathologists attached to medical institutions, in which the volume of surgical specimens is low.

Note on statistical data presented in this eBook:

The senior author (ARC) has been a practicing consultant surgical pathologist for the last 44 years (1969-2013). As a surgical pathologist, he has been associated with 'surgical pathology center' (his own lab), and also attached to the following hospitals in Mumbai (Bombay): Sir H N Hospital, Bombay Hospital and Jaslok Hospital (all corporate institutions), Bone Registry, Grant Medical College; Cytology department of KEM Hospital.

He has gathered vast amount of neoplastic cases of different organ-systems and the data has been in the form of Tables. The tabulation of tumors has been based on classification of anatomical site and behavior (benign, intermediate or malignant). This is not purported to be a population based epidemiological data. However, the data likely represents a fair cross sectional distribution and representation of various neoplasms in the population served in Metropolitan Mumbai (Bombay), India.

DISCLAIMER:

This Book titled Diagnostic Problems in Tumors of Bone: Selected topics, is made available by the Authors solely for trained and licensed physician for personal, non-commercial teaching and educational use. No two individual patients with neoplasms are identical and therefore diagnosis and treatment varies greatly depending on the medical and surgical history. The information contained in this Book is not medical advice. It is the professional responsibility of the practitioner to apply the information provided in a specific situation. Attention has been taken for accuracy of the information presented to describe generally accepted practices; however, knowledge and best practice in the field constantly change with new research. Readers are advised to check the most current information. The authors, editors and publishers are not responsible for errors or omissions or for any outcomes from the use of the information in this book and make no warranty, expressed or implied, with respect to the currency, completeness or accuracy of the content of the publication. This educational application is not a medical device and does not and should not be construed to provide health related or medical advice, or clinical decision support or to support or replace the diagnosis, recommendation, advise, treatment or decision by an appropriately trained licensed physician, including, without limitation with respect to any life sustaining or lifesaving treatment or decision. This educational material does not create a physician patient relationship between the authors and any individual. Before making any medical or health related decision, individuals, including those with any neoplasms are advised to consult an appropriately trained and licensed physician. To the fullest extent of the law, the authors, the editors or the publisher do not assume any liability for any injury and/or damage to persons or property arising out of or related to any use of the material contained in this book.

Chapter 1: Introduction and Classification

Bone tumors are uncommon. Bone tumors are treated on regular basis in selected hospitals only. Hence many general pathologists are not conversant with histological nuances of these tumors. The present attempt is to introduce and initiate postgraduate students and practicing surgical pathologists to this interesting area of diagnostic pathology.

There are about six dozen primary bone tumors and tumor-like lesions, of which 20 are benign tumors and about three dozen are malignant tumors. Metastatic tumors in bone form sizeable portion, though only a small number of these present clinically as primary bone tumors. In addition, there are 18 tumor-like lesions including cysts, reactive lesions and metabolic diseases which may initially present as isolated space occupying swellings mimicking primary bone tumors. As a first step, bone tumors are to be differentiated from non-neoplastic tumor-like lesions, a challenging task for a general surgical pathologist not used to seeing these lesions regularly.

Great advances have been made in therapy and management of bone tumors in the last three decades. Outlook for patients with malignant bone tumors (majority occurring in young individuals), has greatly improved. The scene is not as dismal as it once used to be. In this improved scenario, precise histological diagnosis and classification is of paramount importance. Imaging studies form an important aspect in the diagnosis of bone tumors. As bone tumors have predilection for different age groups, different bones and different parts of a bone (epiphysis, metaphysis and diaphysis), precise localization of the lesion becomes the first step. Next step is to assess the nature of the lesion on the basis of margins, extent of the tumor, presence or absence of sclerotic margins etc. While benign tumors show well delineated margins which are sometimes sclerotic, malignant tumors show ill-defined, infiltrative margins. Infective process is also a destructive lesion, and not uncommonly differentiating infective process from malignant lesion becomes difficult or even impossible on imaging studies.

Before histological diagnosis is established, the pathologist is advised to look at the X rays and other imaging studies to consider possible and probable diagnoses. Still better would be to understand the imaging studies in consultation with a radiologist with special interest in bone tumors. Discussion with the clinician would reveal the history and clinical examination findings. However, it is necessary to emphasize that in the end, it is the Pathologist's responsibility to make the final diagnosis based mainly on histological findings, notwithstanding discrepant radiological features.

Bone tumors are classified according to the matrix they produce. Tumors that produce cartilage or bone or combination of these two elements, form the major bulk of bone tumors.

Benign cartilaginous tumors are far more common than the benign osseous tumors. While malignant osseous tumors are far more common in younger patients, malignant cartilaginous tumors are tumors of older patients and are quite rare in children and younger patients. Another therapeutically significant difference is that osteosarcomas are far more aggressive and metastasize systemically; on the other hand, chondrosarcomas are less aggressive, metastasize infrequently and too late in the course of the disease. High grade conventional osteosarcomas are much more common than the low grade osteosarcomas, and respond favorably to neoadjuvant chemotherapy. In contrast, low grade chondrosarcomas are far more common than the high grade chondrosarcomas, and both types of chondrosarcomas are not responsive to chemotherapy or radiation

Classification of tumors and tumor-like lesions of bone

Cartilaginous tumors:

Benign

Osteochondroma (exostosis):
Solitary osteochondroma
Multiple osteochondromas
Hereditary multiple osteochondromatosis

Reactive osteochondromatous lesions

Bizarre parosteal osteochondromatous proliferation (Nora's lesion)
Tori (osteochondromatous exostoses) of jaws and craniofacial bones
Subungual exostosis
Turret exostosis (Acquired osteochondroma)
Florid reactive periosteitis

Benign intraosseous chondromatous tumors

Enchondroma
Multiple enchondromas
Ollier's disease
Maffucci syndrome
Chondrodysplasia
Periosteal (juxta-cortical) chondroma
Chondroblastoma
Chondromyxoid fibroma
Synovial chondromatosis

Malignant cartilaginous tumors

Primary (intra-osseous) chondrosarcoma
Secondary chondrosarcoma
Periosteal (juxta-articular) chondrosarcoma
Dedifferentiated chondrosarcoma
Clear cell chondrosarcoma
Mesenchymal chondrosarcoma
Skeletal myxoid chondrosarcoma (Parachordomas)

Osseous tumors:

Benign

Ivory osteoma (cranial)
Surface (juxta cortical) osteoma of long bones

Bone Island
Osteoid osteoma
Osteoblastoma
Epithelioid multinodular osteoblastomas

Malignant osseous tumors:
Intramedullary

High grade conventional osteosarcoma
Osteoblastic
Chondroblastic
Fibroblastic
Giant cell rich
Epithelioid cell
Telangiectatic osteosarcoma
Small cell osteosarcoma
Low grade intra-osseous osteosarcoma
Osteoblastoma-like osteosarcoma
Chondroblastoma-like osteosarcoma
Osteosarcoma of jaws
Secondary osteosarcoma

Surface

Parosteal osteosarcoma
Dedifferentiated parosteal osteosarcoma
Periosteal osteosarcoma
High grade surface osteosarcoma

Fibro-osseous lesions:

Fibrous dysplasia, solitary
Multiple fibrous dysplasias
McCune –Albright syndrome
Osteofibrous dysplasia
Fibrocartilaginous mesenchymoma

Fibrous lesions:

Benign

Metaphyseal fibrous defect (Non-ossifying fibroma)
Multifocal metaphyseal fibrous defect (Jaffe-Campanacci syndrome)
Benign fibrous histiocytoma
Fibromyxoma / myxoma
Juvenile multifocal myofibromatosis
Desmoplastic fibroma (locally aggressive)

Malignant

Fibrosarcoma
Undifferentiated high grade pleomorphic sarcoma (Malignant fibrous histiocytoma) (so called)

Giant cell lesions:
Benign

Giant cell reparative granuloma (solid aneurysmal bone cyst)
Brown tumor of hyperparathyroidism

Potentially malignant

Giant cell tumor (osteoclastoma) of bone

Malignant

Malignant giant cell tumor ("de novo" or secondary)

Round cell tumors:

Ewing sarcoma / PNET
Adamantinoma like Ewing sarcoma
Malignant lymphoma
Plasma cell myeloma (solitary and multiple)
Granulocytic sarcoma

Histiocytic tumors:

Langerhans cell histiocytosis
Rosai-Dorfman disease
Erdheim Chester disease

Vascular tumors:
Benign

Hemangioma
Angiomatosis
Lymphangioma
Glomus tumor
Gorham's lesion (massive osteolysis)

Malignant

Epithelioid hemangioendothelioma (Intermediate grade malignant)
Hemangiopericytoma
Angiosarcoma / Malignant hemangioendothelioma
Kaposi's sarcoma

Neural tumors:
Benign

Schwannoma

Malignant
>   Malignant peripheral nerve sheath tumor

Lipomatous tumors:

Benign
>   Lipoma

Malignant
>   Liposarcoma

Cysts:

Benign
>   Solitary (simple/ unicameral) bone cyst
>   Aneurysmal bone cyst
>   Ganglion cyst
>   Epidermal cyst

Miscellaneous:

>   Adamantinoma
>   Ewing-like adamantinoma
>   Benign Notochordal cell tumor
>   Chordoma / Chondroid chordoma

Metastatic malignant tumors

Diseases which may mimic bone tumors

>   Infections
>   Fracture callus
>   Myositis ossificans
>   Avulsive cortical irregularity / periosteal desmoid
>   Radiation injury

Table 1: Malignant tumors of bone (Dr. Arun Chitale, Data from Bone registry, Grant Medical College, Mumbai)	
Giant cell tumor (locally invasive tumor)	639 (21.66%)
Malignant giant cell tumor	26 (0.88%)
Metastatic malignancy (over 99% carcinomas)	635 (21.53%)
Osteogenic sarcoma	555 (18.81%)
Plasma cell myeloma	257 (8.71%)
Solitary plasmacytoma	14 (0.47%)
Ewing sarcoma/PNET	244 (8.27%)
Chondrosarcoma	225 (7.63%)
Lymphoma	127 (4.31%)
Desmoplastic fibroma (locally invasive)	63 (2.14%)
Fibrosarcoma	62 (2.10%)
Undifferentiated malignant bone tumor (MFH)	50 (1.69%)
Chordoma	41 (1.39%)
Epithelioid hemangioendothelioma	6 (0.20%)
Angiosarcoma	3 (0.10%)
Miscellaneous sarcomas; (MPNST, Liposarcoma, Leiomyosarcoma (one each)	3 (0.10%)
Total	2950 (100.00%)

Table 2: Benign tumor and tumor-like lesions of bone (Dr. Arun Chitale, Data from Bone registry, Grant Medical College, and Surgical Pathology Center, Mumbai)	
Osteochondroma	489 (30.4%)
Multiple osteochondromatosis	20 (1.2%)
Enchondroma (chondroma)	187 (11.6%)
Multiple enchondromatosis	3 (0.2%)
Chondroblastoma	113 (7.0%)
Chondromyxoid fibroma	33 (2.0%)
Osteoma	16 (1.0%)
Osteoid osteoma	124 (7.7%)
Osteoblastoma	10 (0.6%)
Fibrous dysplasia	274 (17.0%)
Polyostotic fibrous dysplasia	14 (0.9%)
Non-ossifying fibroma	78 (4.8%)
Unicameral bone cyst	295 (18.3%)
Aneurysmal bone cyst	159 (9.9%)
Total	1611 (100.0%)

Chapter 2: Cartilaginous tumors

Osteochondroma (Exostosis)

Osteochondroma (exostosis) is the most common bone tumor. It presents as a knobby or mushroom-like bony projections with or without a stalk. It has cartilage cap on the surface of the bone that recapitulates structure of normal articular end of bone. It has medullary cavity and cortex; and both are continuous with those of the underlying host bone. In an excised specimen of osteochondroma it is not possible to demonstrate this continuity of the cortex and medulla with those of the underlying bone (Fig. 1A, B, C, D). Hence strictly speaking, definitive diagnosis of osteochondroma is possible only on imaging studies. This key feature of osteochondroma differentiates it from other similar osteochondromatous lesions on the surface of the bone. These include bizarre parosteal osteochondromatous proliferation (BPOP or Nora's lesion), parosteal osteosarcoma and several reactive lesions with superficial resemblance to osteochondroma.

Osteochondromas involve any bone that develops through endochondral ossification. These tumors occur more frequently on the surface of long tubular bones, in the metaphyseal and diaphyseal regions. Flat bones like scapula and ilium are also affected though less frequently. Small tubular bones of hands and feet, ribs, jaws and vertebral bones are rarely involved. Craniofacial bones are never involved by osteochondromas.

Majority of osteochondromas occur as solitary tumors. Many remain asymptomatic and even when clinically apparent may not be excised. About 15% occur as autosomal dominant hereditary multiple osteochondromas syndrome. Schmale et al (1994)[1] estimated the incidence of multiple osteochondromas syndrome in general population to be approximately one in 50000.

Radiologic diagnosis of osteochondroma should present no problem, if the criterion of continuity of the cortex and medulla with those of host bone is applied strictly (Fig. 1 A, B).

Grossly this is a nodular mass of cancellous bone covered with cartilaginous cap (Fig. 1 C).

Essentially the tumor is composed of three layers: a) the outermost thin layer of perichondrium; b) cap of hyaline cartilage similar to growth plate, and c) trabecular bone formed by endochondral ossification of hyaline cartilage. Characteristically in the center of osteochondroma there is medullary cavity that is continuous with that of the underlying bone, as emphasized earlier. Osteochondroma does not contain spindle cell component, unlike bizarre parosteal osteochondromatous proliferation (Nora's lesion)

Surgical excision proves curative in most cases. In the Mayo Clinic series[2] 2% of the osteochondromas recurred. Recurrence may be attributed to incomplete surgical removal. At least in a few cases recurrence of so called osteochondroma raises doubt if original lesion was indeed low grade chondrosarcoma misinterpreted as osteochondroma.

Rarely secondary chondrosarcoma may develop on osteochondroma. True incidence of this phenomenon is difficult to estimate. The Mayo Clinic series[2] reports an incidence of secondary chondrosarcomas in 8.5 % of surgically excised solitary osteochondromas. In a study of 107 secondary chondrosarcomas, 61 patients had solitary osteochondroma, and 46 had multiple osteochondromas. 5-

and 10-year mortality rate was 1.6% and 4.8% respectively. Five patients died of metastatic disease and others of local rcurrences[3].

Secondary chondrosarcoma is suspected when the original lesion becomes large and painful. Radiologically there is marked thickening and irregularity with lucent areas in the cartilage cap. Infiltration of the tumor in the soft tissue confirms diagnosis of malignancy.

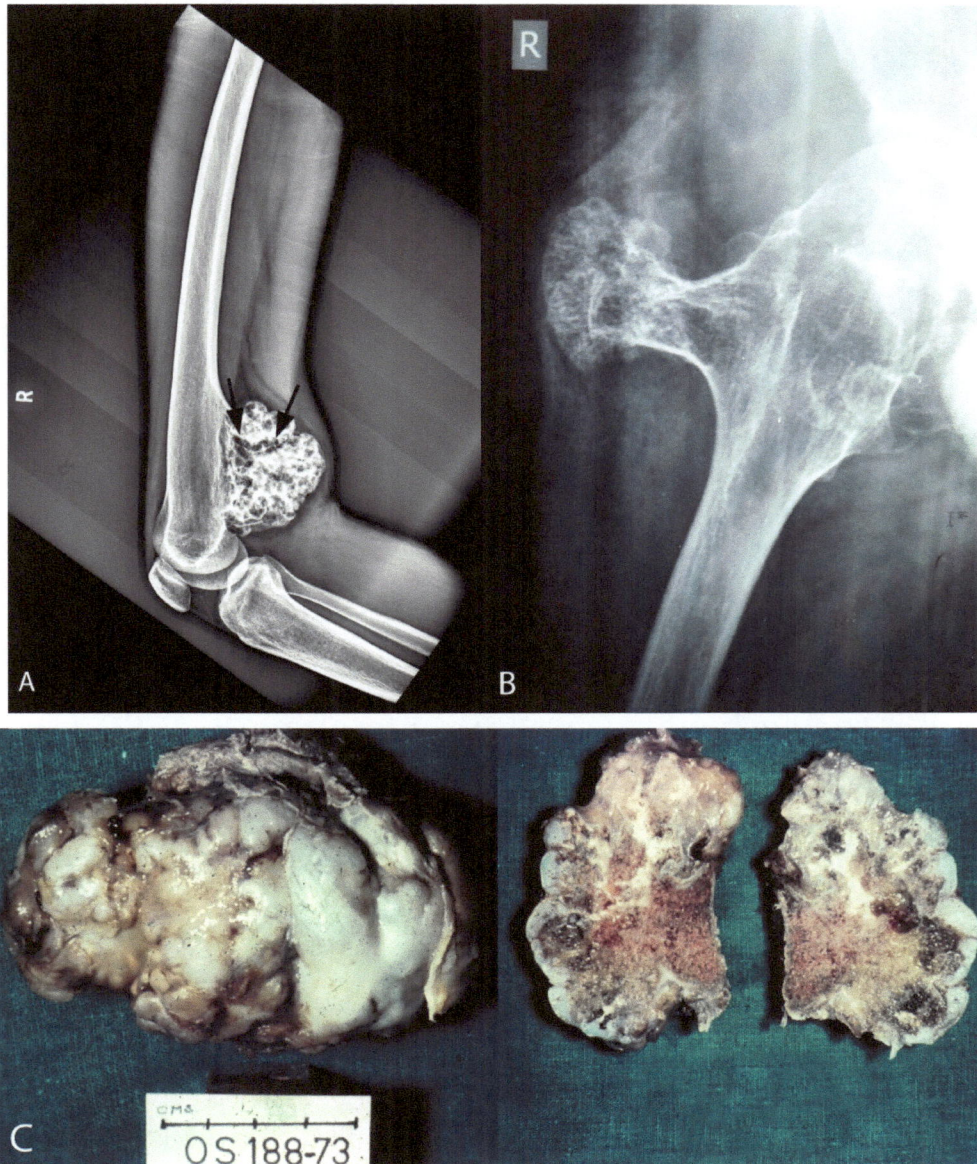

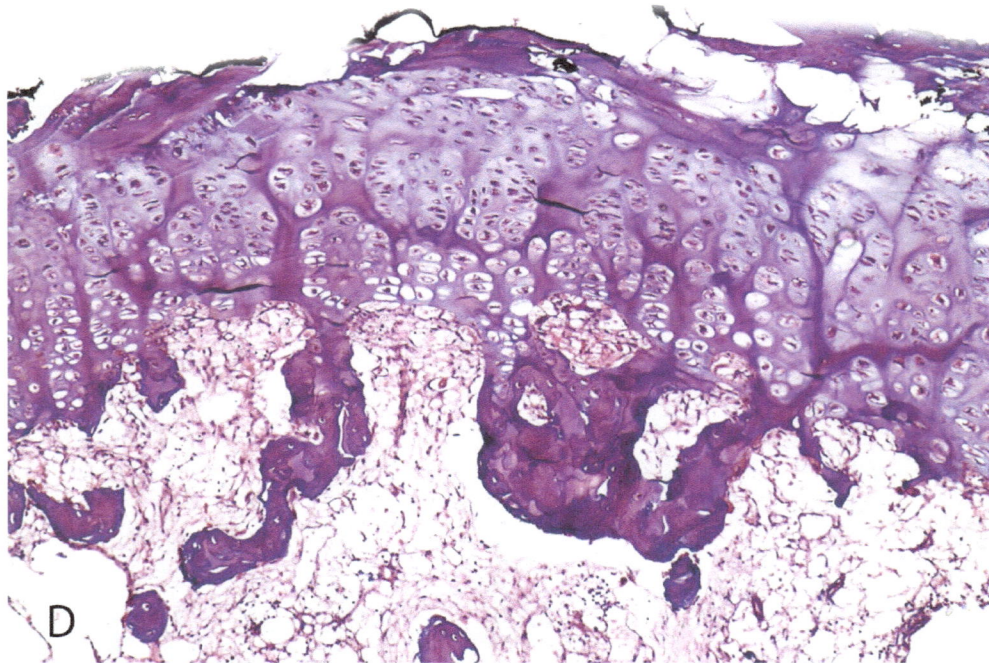

Fig.2.1 (A) X ray of knee joint showing bony out growth arising from the lower end of the femur, arrows show continuity of medullary cavity; (B) Osteochondroma: upper end of femur: medullary cavity within osteochondroma is in continuity with that of femur; (C) Osteochondroma in a case of multiple osteochondromatosis; (D) Scanner view of osteochondroma: thick plate of hyaline cartilage overlying a mass of cancellous bone with fatty marrow.

Bizarre parosteal osteochondromatous proliferation (B - POP) / Nora's lesion

Nora and colleagues first reported this lesion in 1983 as reactive 'bizarre osteocartilaginous and spindle cell proliferation' on the surface of small bones of hands and feet that could be mistaken for malignancy by the unwary. It is now realized that almost half the cases occur on the surface of long tubular bones [4, 5, 6]

Radiologically the lesion appears as an osteocartilaginous mass firmly adherent to the cortex (Fig. 2 A).

Grossly this is nodular cartilaginous mass adherent to the cortex (Fig. 2 B)

The basic structure of B POP consists of cartilaginous proliferation with maturation in to woven or lamellar bone, and spindle cell proliferation around the cartilage and in the intertrabecular spaces (Fig. 2 C & D). Characteristically the bone trabeculae show deep blue or purple staining earlier thought to be almost pathognomonic of the lesion. It is now realized that similar deep purple staining of bone occurs in many other situations, both reactive and neoplastic.

Almost half the cases of bizarre parosteal osteochondromatous proliferations especially those that occur on long tubular bones recur, and 20 % recurred more than once. The lesion may simulate osteosarcoma [7] and chromosomal abnormalities have been described in some of these cases.

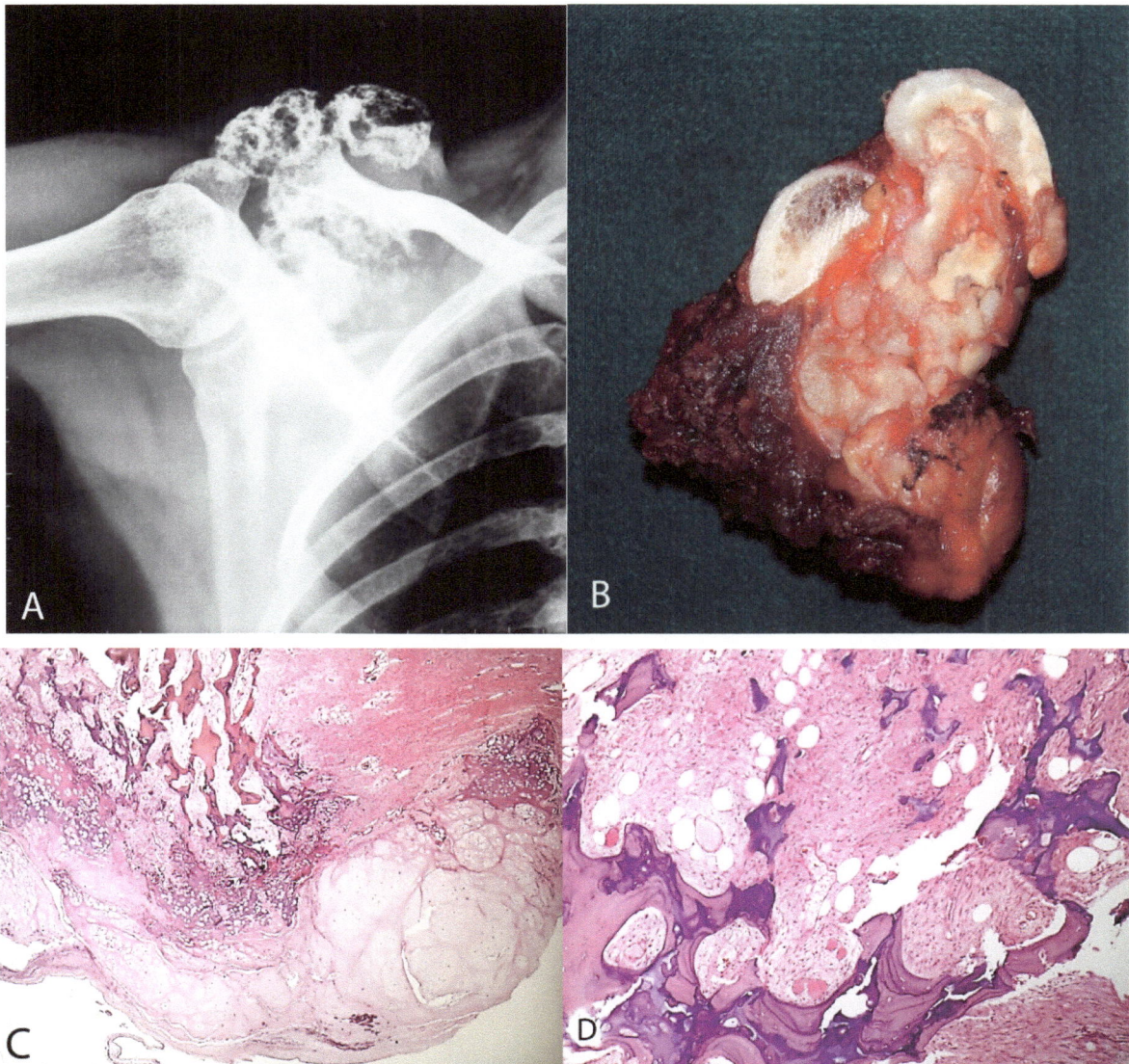

Fig.2.2 Bizarre parosteal osteochondromatous proliferation (BPOP/ Nora's lesion) X ray of shoulder joint showing large osteocartilaginous mass; (B) BPOP- A large multinodular osteocartilaginous mass on the surface, adherent to the cortex; (C) BPOP which is made up of cartilage, bone and spindle cells; (D) spindle cell proliferation and deep purple discoloration of the bone are distinguishing features of BPOP; may remotely resemble parosteal osteosarcoma.

Another lesion which may resemble B POP is parosteal osteosarcoma which also may exhibit the same three structural components: namely cartilage, bone and spindle cells. B POP, however, is predominantly a chondroid lesion while parosteal osteosarcoma is predominantly osseous and spindle cellular. Conceptually speaking, since 50 % of the B POP occurring on the surface of the long tubular bones recurs, and several show chromosomal abnormalities, it may be tempting to postulate that B Pop may be related to parosteal osteosarcoma.

Reactive osteochondromatous lesions on the surface of bone:

There are several types of reactive lesions that occur on the surface of bone, mostly on the small bones of hands and feet that present as primary bone tumors[8]. Most are related to some injury, and generally resemble myositis ossificans. Histology varies according to duration. In early stage, histologic features are often mistaken for malignancy. Generally, these show cartilaginous, osseous and fibroblastic/myofibroblastic proliferation in varying proportions. As in myositis ossificans there is zonal maturation. The reactive lesions are self-limiting, and mature into regularly arranged trabeculae. The various entities are: florid reactive periosteitis (Fig 3A &B), turret (acquired) osteochondroma, subungual exostosis, torus, exostosis of the jaw and cranial bones, and aural meatal exostosis.

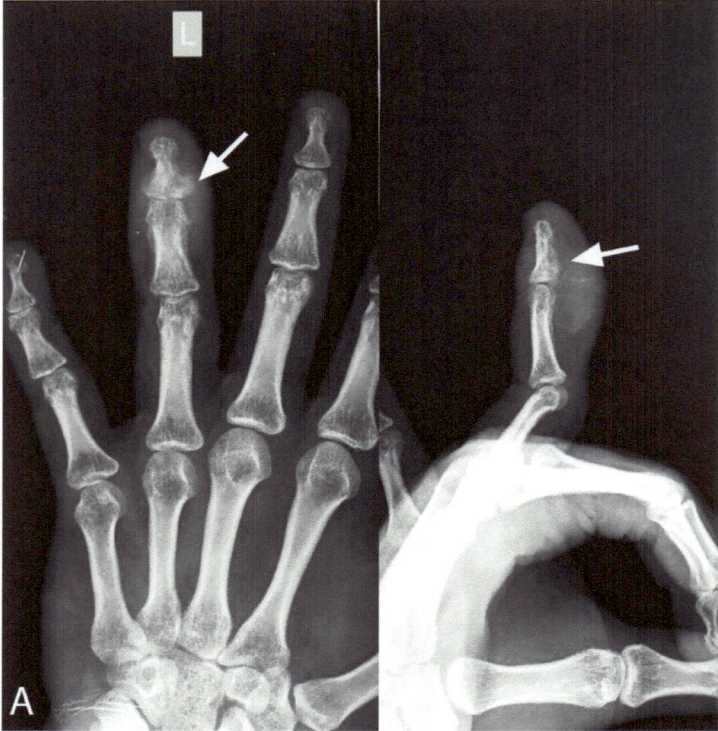

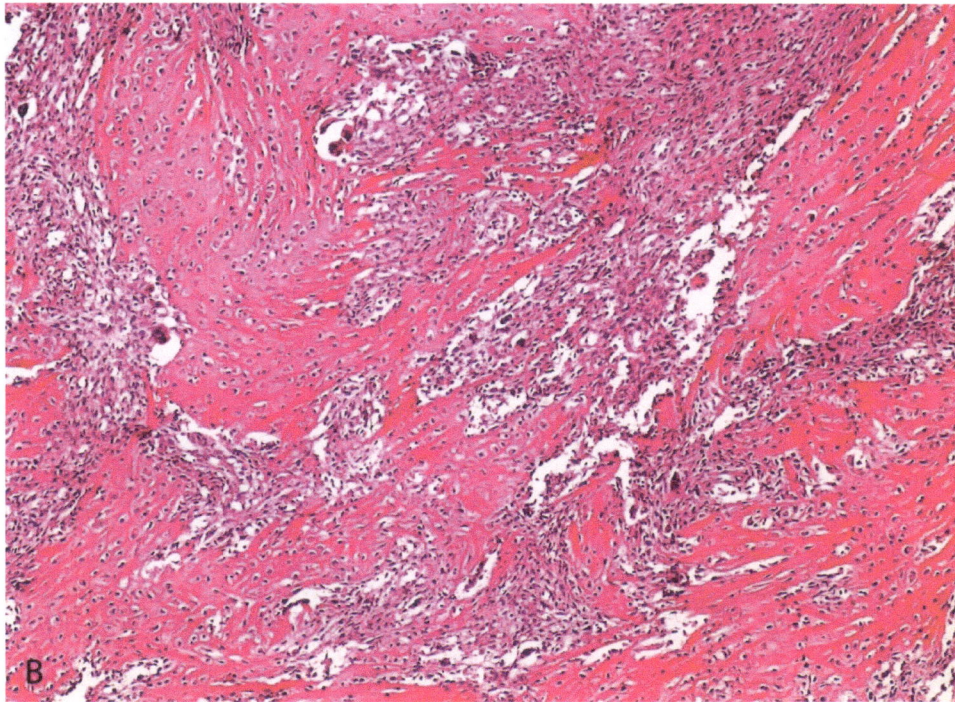

Fig.2.3 A) Periosteitis of terminal phalanx of ring finger; B) Reactive changes including fibrosis, focal vascularity, inflammatory cells and osteoid.

Periosteal chondroma

Periosteal chondroma (Fig A, B), like enchondroma, is a benign cartilaginous tumor that occurs mainly in young individuals However, unlike enchondroma, periosteal chondroma occurs on the surface of bone, and involves long tubular bones. Increased cellularity, nuclear atypia and binucleation may occur in benign periosteal chondroma, and are not reliable features to differentiate between benign and malignant lesions[9]. In a study of 46 peripheral chondromas, the tumor is found to be a small well-marginated, nodule with cortical erosion but no invasion. Parosteal chondrosarcoma presents as a nodular mass involving the cortex. Arbitrarily periosteal cartilaginous tumors that are less than 5 cm in its largest diameter are considered as benign lesions even when they show mild nuclear atypia and increased cellularity; and those that are larger than 5 cm are taken as grade 1 chondrosarcomas[10].

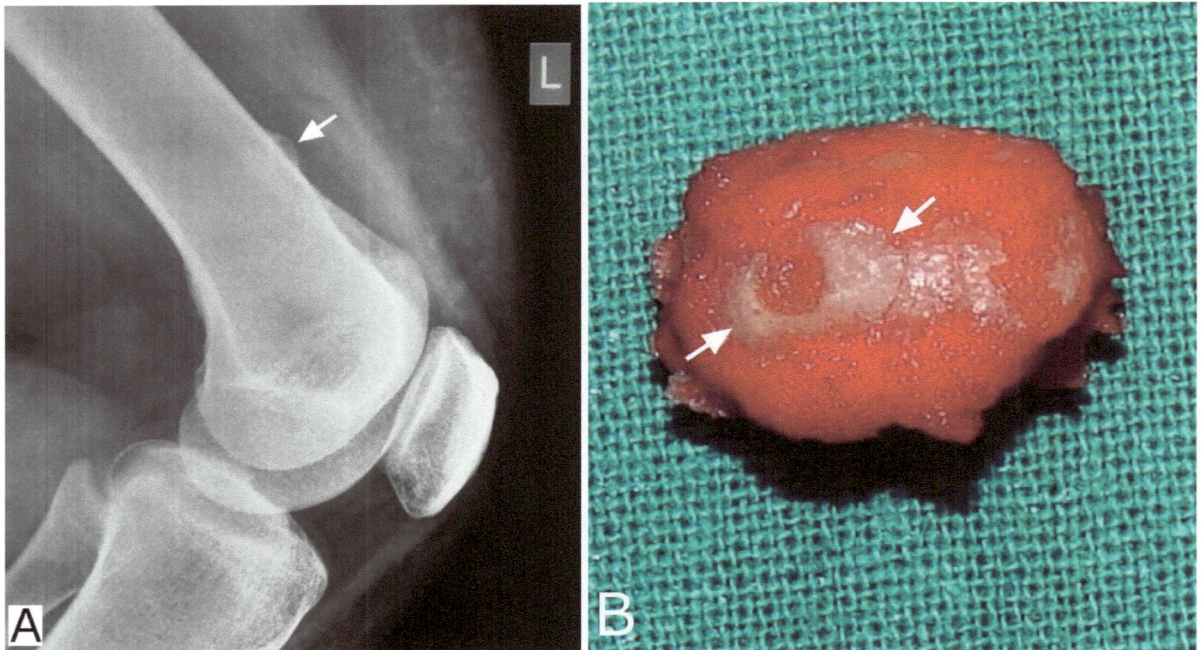

Fig 2.4 Periosteal chondroma: (A) Oval, smooth, translucent bubble-like periosteal over growth (arrow); (B) widely excised nodule, note the biopsy defect seen within pale grey lesion (arrows) and broad surrounding normal host tissue.

Enchondroma

Enchondroma are benign cartilaginous tumors that occur in the medullary cavity of bones. Short tubular bones of hands and feet are the common sites of involvement accounting for 40 % of the cases; long tubular bones particularly proximal humerus and proximal and distal femur are next in frequency. Enchondromas in bones of hand and feet are more cellular and atypical than those of long bones; these should not be mistaken for low grade chondrosarcoma. Flat bones like scapula, pelvis, sternum, and vertebrae are rarely involved. Almost all the cases of cartilage tumors that occur in sternum are malignant.

A small proportion of enchondromas are multiple, often unilaterally. The cases of multiple enchondromatosis are called 'Ollier's disease', named after Louis Xavier Edouard Leopold Olliere, a French orthopaedic surgeon who first recognized a case of multiple enchondromas in a six-year-old girl in 1897.Almost 25 to 30 % of patients with Ollier's diseases develop secondary chondrosarcomas in one of the enchondromas.

Multiple enchondroma associated with soft tissue angioma is known as 'Maffucci's syndrome', named after Angelo Maria Maffucci (1847–1903), an Italian Pathologist at University of Pisa who first described this association. Malignant transformation in these patients is estimated to be higher than that in Ollier's disease. Solitary enchondromas that occur in short tubular bones of hands and feet may be either asymptomatic, or present with pain. Some cause expansion of bone and may result in fracture. Those occurring in long tubular bones are often asymptomatic, and are recognized incidentally.

Enchondromas that occur in short tubular bones of hands and feet may be well marginated and show lucent or less commonly mineralized appearance (Fig. 5 A, B, C).

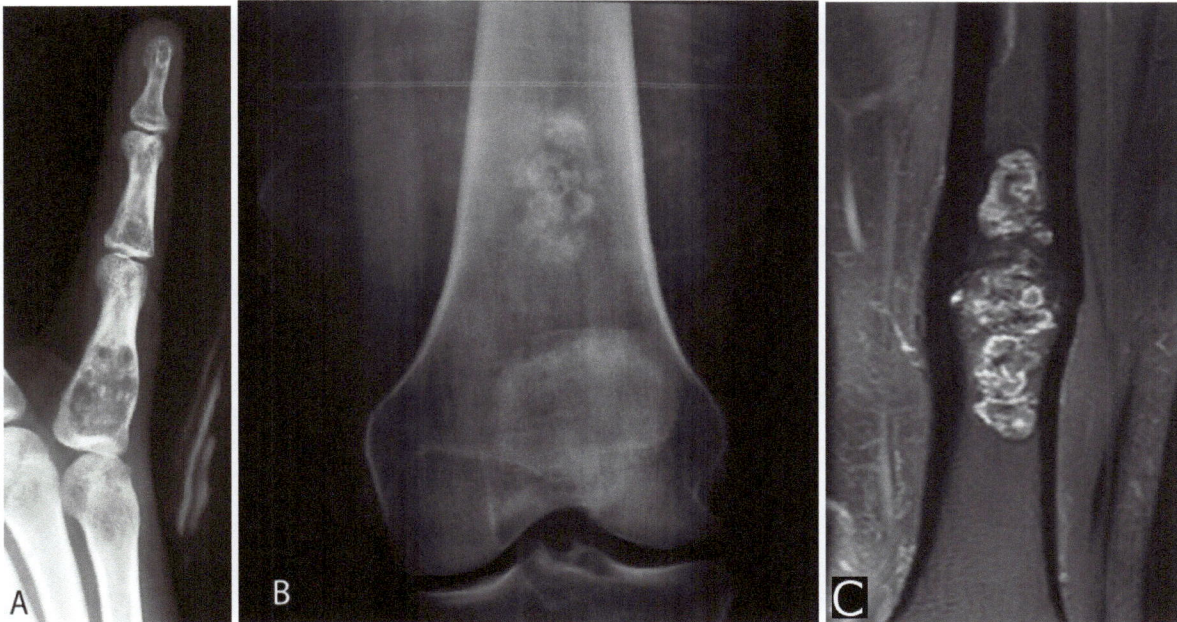

Fig. 2.5 (A) Enchondroma of the proximal phalanx of the little finger; (B) Enchondroma at the lower metaphysis of the femur with cartilage calcification- rings and arcs; (C) low grade chondrosarcoma in midshaft of femur

Some tumors may cause expansion of bone and result in fracture with extension to soft tissue, which should not be interpreted as evidence of malignancy. Enchondromas of long tubular bones are predominantly medullary without erosion of the endosteum. Endosteal erosion, cortical thickening and bone expansion should raise suspicion of malignancy.

Gross appearance of enchondromas is rather characteristic: nodular, firm, pearly white, opalescent and gritty with areas of calcification and ossification.

Microscopic

The lesion appears multinodular and composed of hypocellular and avascular hyaline cartilage with calcification. Hyaline cartilage often shows rim of lamellar bone. Normal marrow tissue of host bone may be seen in between the nodules. In case of short tubular bones, focal myxoid change, increased cellularity, double nuclei, enlargement of nuclei and prominent nucleoli may be present and should not be interpreted as evidence of malignancy (Fig.6 A, B, C, D). Destruction of bone with extension of tumor in the soft tissue in the absence of fracture is the only reliable evidence of malignancy.

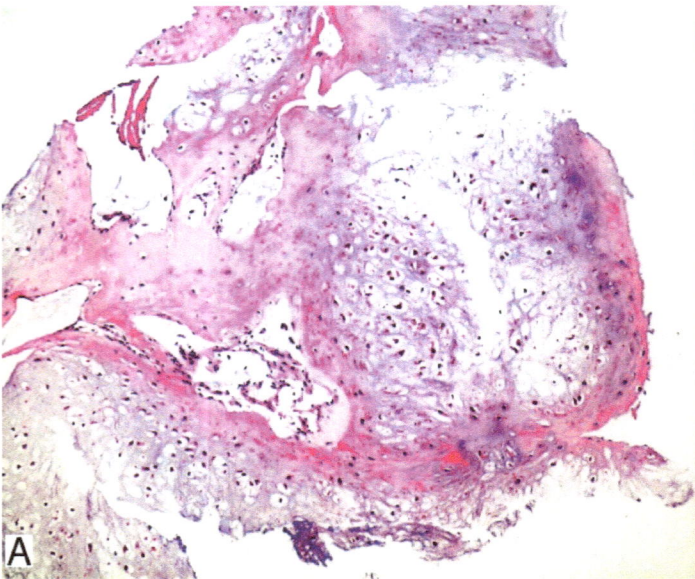
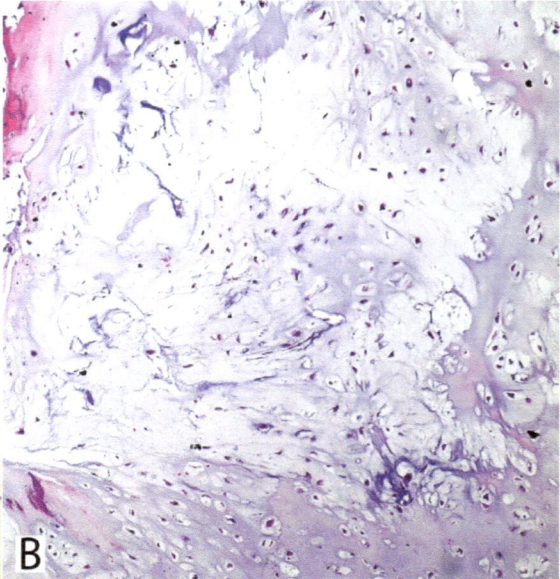

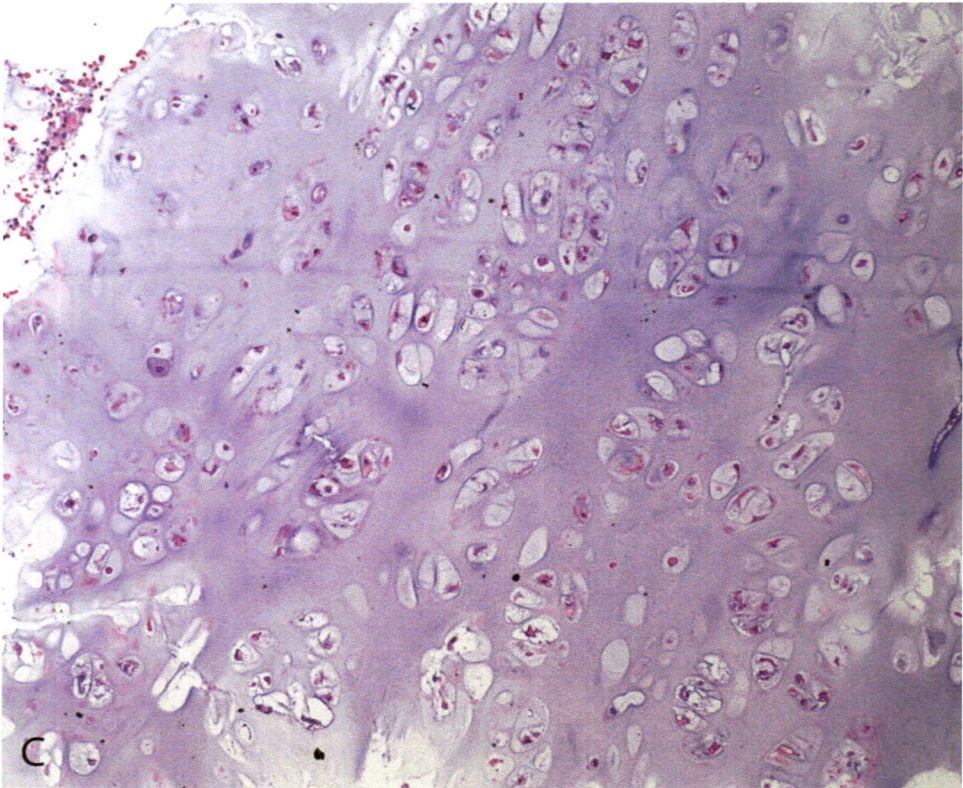

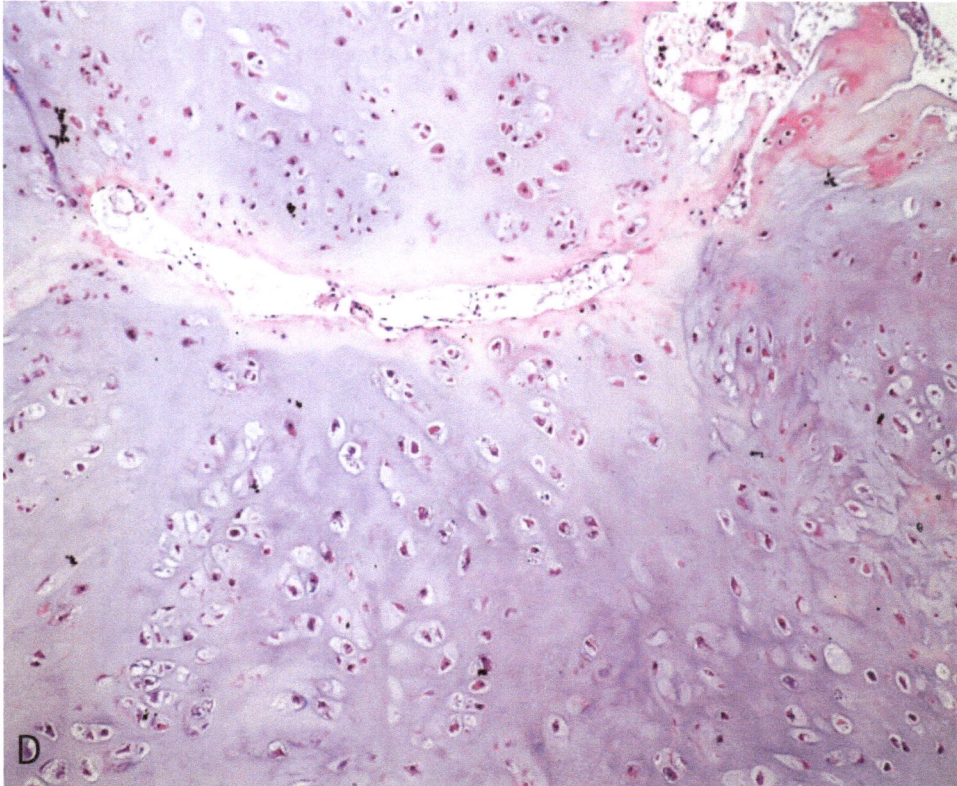

Fig. 2.6: Enchondroma (A) note the peripheral rim of ossification; (B, C, D) these are various faces of enchondroma; note excess cellularity but the lesion is benign.

Prognosis

Enchondromas of long tubular bones, particularly in adults, pose a difficult problem. Pain, expansion of bone, endosteal erosion, cortical thickening and myxoid change should raise suspicion of malignancy. Tumors of short tubular bones are most often benign, and malignancy should be diagnosed with care. On the other hand, cartilage tumors in long tubular bones are more often malignant, and in this group benign lesions should be diagnosed with care. In both situations differentiating between enchondromas from grade 1 chondrosarcomas should not be based solely on histological features.

Chondroblastoma

Emory Codman (1931) first segregated this tumor from a group of giant cell containing epiphyseal tumors and called its epiphyseal chondromatous giant cell tumor', hence the eponym 'Codman's tumor[10]. It is a tumor of adolescents and young persons (age group 10-25 years). There is a male predominance. The lesion attracts clinical attention because of pain and restriction of movements. About75% of the chondroblastomas occurs in the epiphysis of long tubular bones; mainly in distal and proximal femur, proximal humerus and proximal tibia. Flat bones such as acetabulum and ilium are also involved. Talus, calcaneum and patella are rare sites of involvement. Exceptionally cranio-facial bones are involved

On x-ray, this is a well demarcated, small, lucent lesion with sclerotic border, about 2-5cm in size and typically located in the epiphysis. The tumor is usually not expansile and about 30% may show matrix calcification (Fig. 7 A, B).

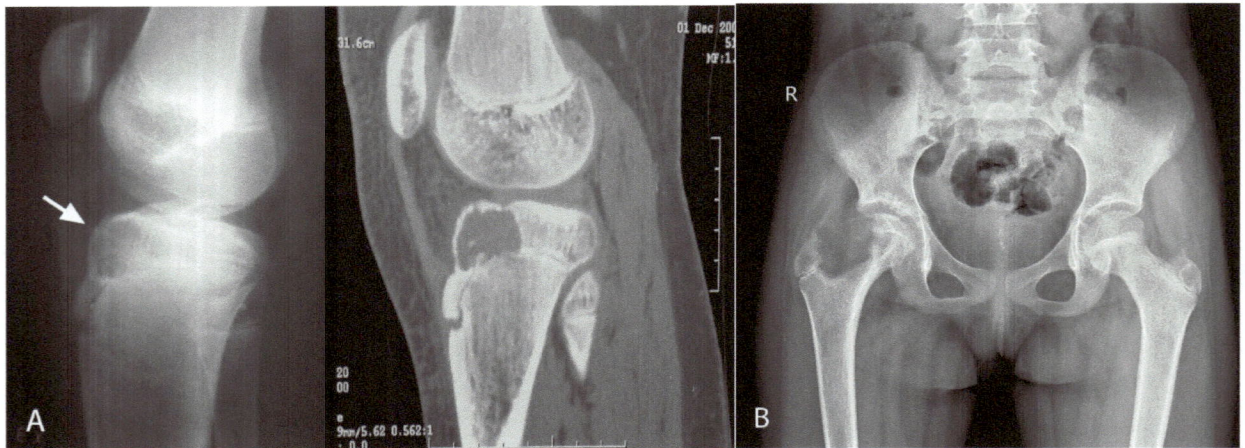

Fig. 2.7 Benign epiphyseal chondroblastoma A) x-ray & CT picture of tibia with a lytic lesion restricted to the epiphysis; (B) X ray of a large chondroblastoma of femoral head (right), transgressing part of epiphyseal plate and causing destruction of sub epiphyseal bone and trochanter.

Gross

The tumor is gritty brownish white and almost fills the epiphysis. It often shows cysts and in some cases superimposed by an area of aneurysmal bone cyst.

Microscopic

Chondroblastoma is characterized by nodules of eosinophilic chondroid material surrounded by sheets of oval to spindle shaped chondroblasts with characteristic linear nuclear grooves not unlike those seen in Langerhans cell histiocytosis. The chondroblasts have slightly basophilic cytoplasm with well-defined cytoplasmic borders. Around the individual chondroblasts there is characteristic "chicken wire pattern" of calcification in about 30 % of the cases (Fig 7 C, D, E, F, G). Also seen are areas of floccular calcification in some cases. A fair number of randomly scattered multinucleated giant cells are often seen

Chondroblastomas show secondary aneurysmal bone cyst (ABC) changes in almost 20% of cases. Hence in every case of ABC that occurs at or near the epiphysis, evidence of associated chondroblastoma should be diligently looked for (Fig. 7 H, I, J).

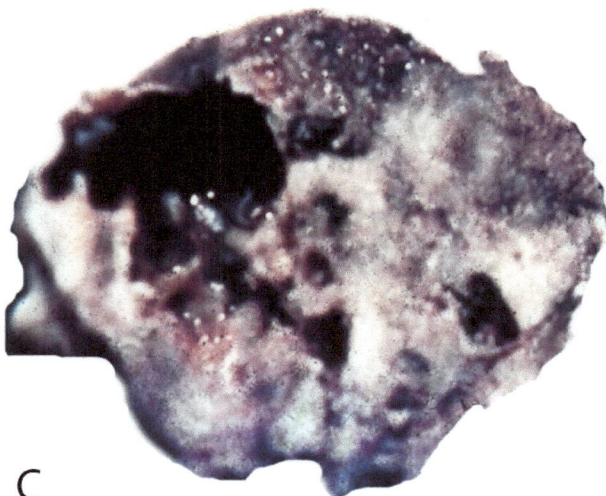

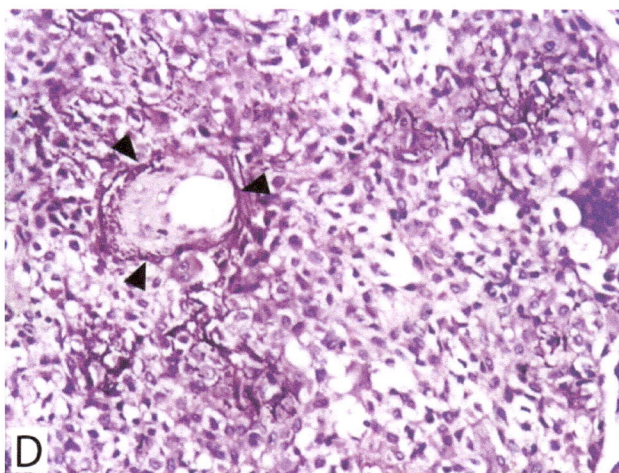

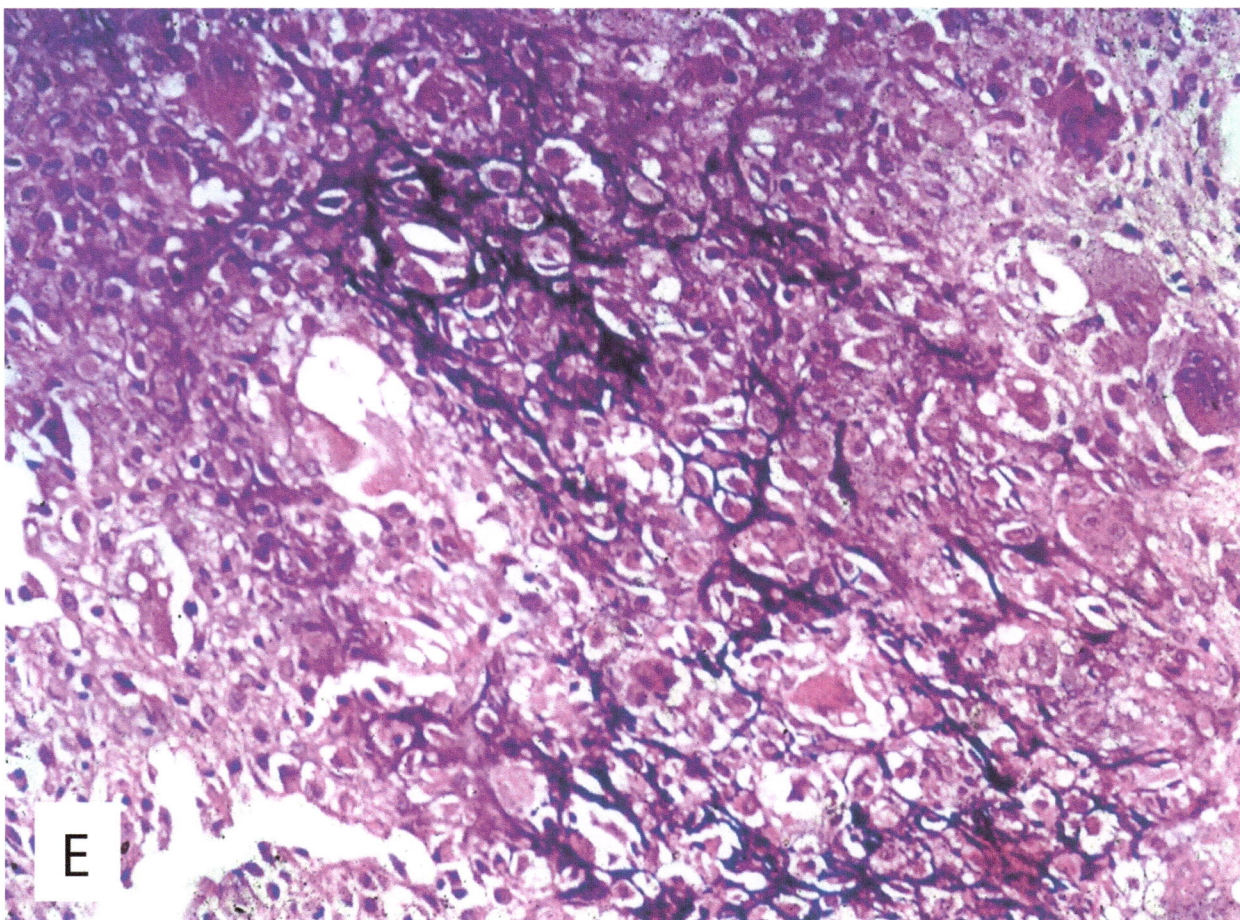

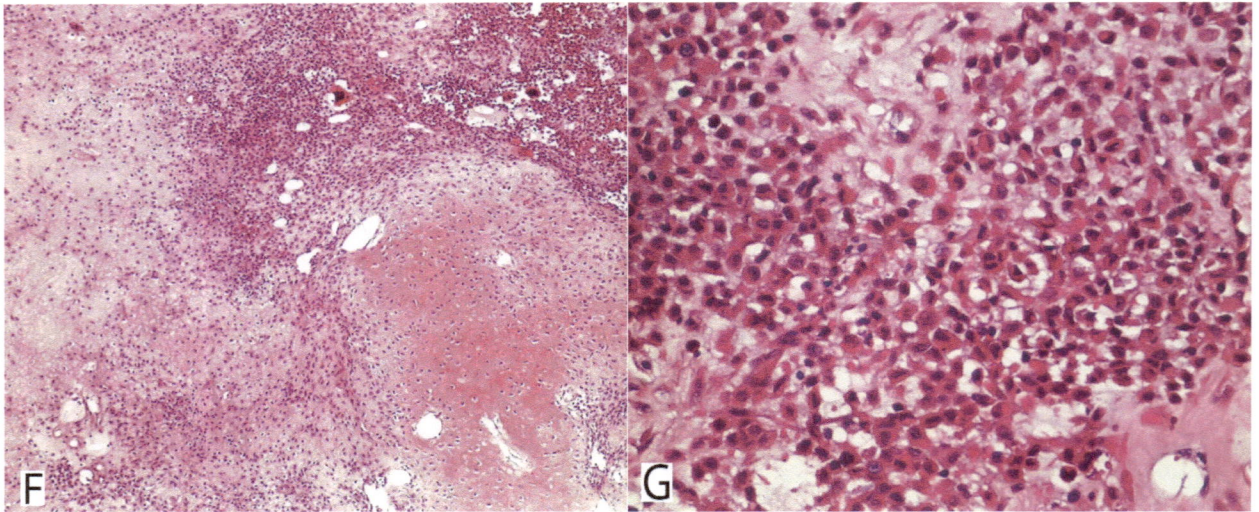

Fig. 2.7 (C) gross appearance of chondroblastoma of humeral head: focally cystic firm whitish tissue; (D) chondroblasts with vacuolated cytoplasm in contiguous sheets, note one small focus of mature cartilage (arrows); (E) "chicken wire" calcification around single or groups of tumor cells; (F) nodule of eosinophilic cartilage (commonly seen) with cellular component of typical eosinophilic chondroblasts; (G) higher magnification of chondroblasts;

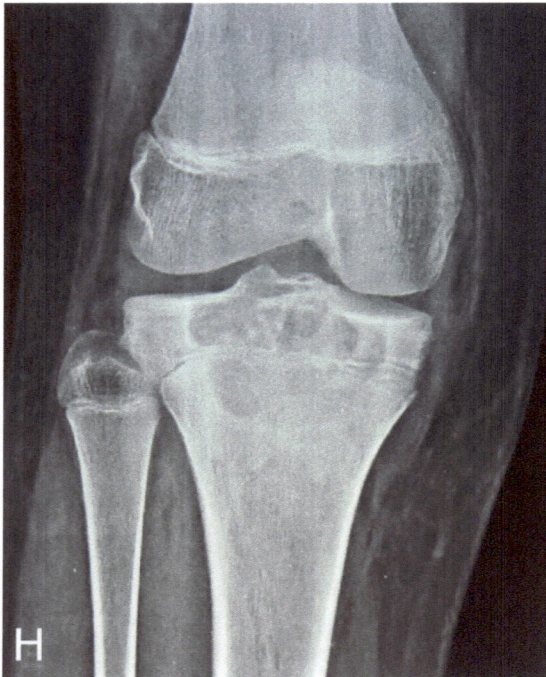

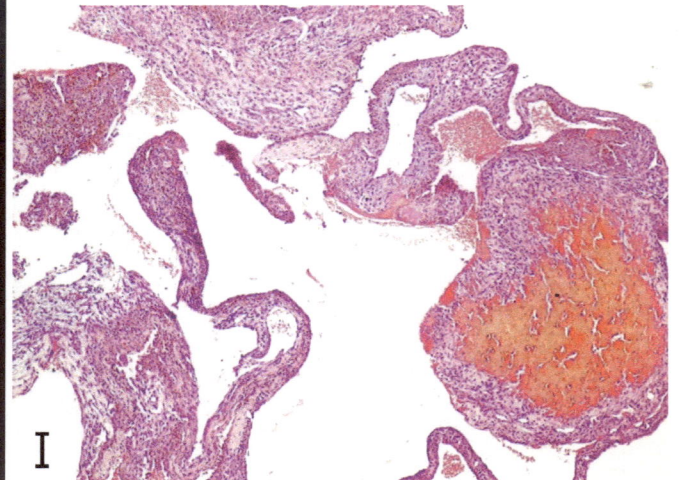

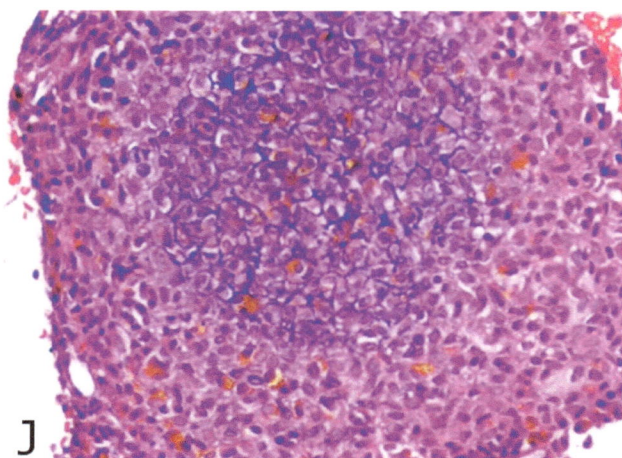

Fig. 2.7 (H) X ray of upper tibia showing chondroblastoma with ABC; (I) ABC component seen in chondroblastoma of tibial epiphysis on x-ray; (J) nodule of chondroblasts in wall of ABC, note lacy calcification

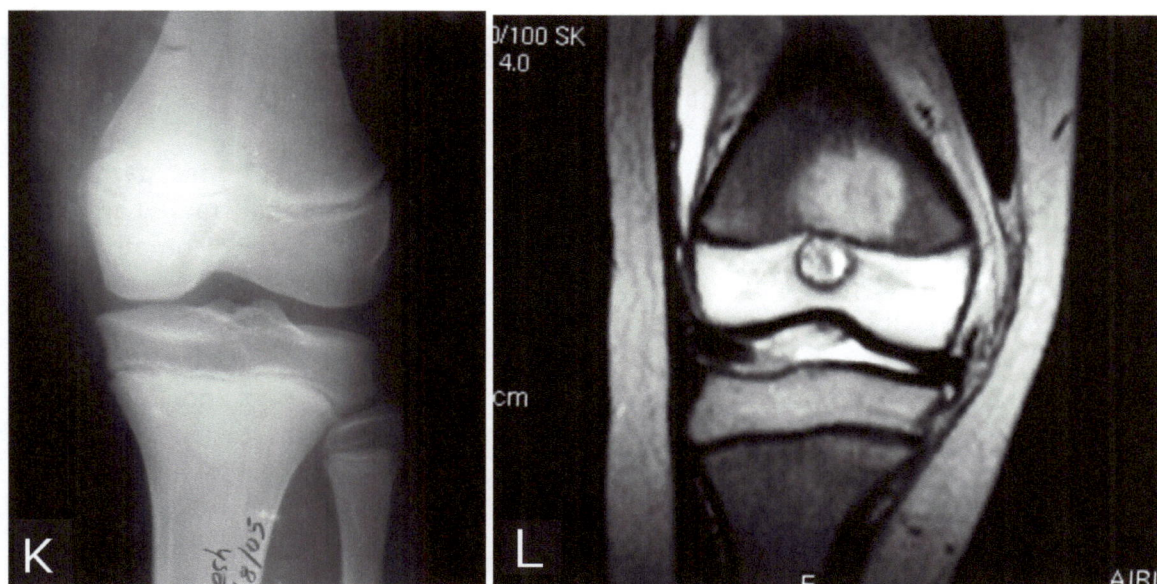

Fig. 2.7 (K) plain x-ray of right knee: no lesion is seen; (L) MRI of the same case reveals well define rounded T2 hyperintense lesion with sclerotic border in the epiphysis of femur, characteristic of chondroblastoma. Note femoral metaphysis shows well defined hyperintense bone marrow edema.

Recurrence and pulmonary metastasis of benign epiphyseal chondroblastoma

The experience of last 70 years or so indicates that curettage with bone packing is curative in most cases of chondroblastoma. Local recurrence can occur after curettage but this is attributed to incomplete curettage or accidental spillage during surgery. Occasionally, these tumors pursue a more aggressive course with invasion of joint spaces and adjacent bones, and exceptionally metastasize [11, 12]. Metastasis in chondroblastoma has not been sufficiently stressed in the literature, unlike metastasis in giant cell tumors. The purpose of this case report is not only to document this uncommon event (the 12th case of lung metastasis) but also to emphasize that patients with chondroblastoma may have metastasis at presentation[13]. The histological characteristics of primary, metastatic, and locally recurrent tumors are identical to those of conventional chondroblastoma. This very unusual feature of histologically benign pulmonary metastasis may be explained as a transport phenomenon, for the following reasons: a) metastasis developed only after surgical therapy; b) only lungs have been involved in all reported cases; c) Some untreated pulmonary metastases have failed to grow and d) metastatectomy has resulted in long-term survival. Examples of "malignant chondroblastoma" may therefore, represent simply a transport phenomenon.

Chondromyxoid fibroma:

Jaffe and Lichtenstein[14] first described this entity cautioning that this is a 'distinctive benign tumor likely to be mistaken for chondrosarcoma'. As Unni and Inwards note, this admonition has been so seriously taken that true chondrosarcomas are being misinterpreted as chondromyxoid fibroma!

Clinical findings

Chondromyxoid fibroma is a rare tumor defined by its benign nature, and characteristic histology. It occurs in the young, the majority being in the second and third decades. There is slight male predominance.

The tumor occurs in the metaphysis of proximal tibia and distal end of femur. Flat bones, particularly ilium, are involved in about 25% of the cases. Small bones of hand and feet, especially tarsals are other sites of involvement. Ribs, vertebrae and facial bones are affected rarely. A large clinico-pathological study of 278 cases of chondromyxoid fibroma showed some more facets of this lesion[15]: periosteal reaction and extension to soft tissues uncommon, excess calcification present in more than 1/3rd of cases and recurrence rate was nearly 25% (no malignant change).

The X-ray (Fig. 8 A) shows lytic, oval, eccentric lesion with scalloped sclerotic borders and is situated in the metaphysis, but may extend in to the epiphysis or diaphysis. In flat bones and short bones of hands and feet the lesions are lucent with no defining features. Grossly the tumor appears white, firm and slightly myxoid. Baker et al[16] reported 20 cases of CMF with juxtacortical location. This lesion tends to occur in ages older than that of conventional central CMF, but enjoys the same benign outcome.

Microscopic

The tumor shows a lobular pattern with a band of condensed spindle fibroblastic/ myofibroblastic cells mixed with multinucleated giant cells at the periphery; while the central portion is hypocellular with stellate or spindle cells embedded in myxoid immature mesenchymal stroma with chondroid differentiation. Hyaline cartilage occurs in about 20 % of the cases (Fig. 8H). Rarely host bone trabeculae may be embedded in the tumor, which should not be taken as evidence of malignancy, unlike in other bone tumors. There may be scattered cells with large hyperchromatic nuclei but mitosis is rare (Fig. 8 B, C, D).

Chondrosarcoma can be differentiated from chondromyxoid fibroma by it's uniformly hypercellular pattern throughout the lobules and more prominent nuclear hyperchromasia and atypia. En block resection is preferred because curetting, if incomplete may result in recurrence. Recurrence rate is estimated to be almost 20%. Clonal arrangements of chromosome 6 with pericentromeric inversion-inv (6) (p25q13) has been consistently found in cases of CMF, and in no other tumor of bones or soft tissues. This cytogenic marker may be useful to differentiate CMF from chondrosarcoma in difficult cases[17].

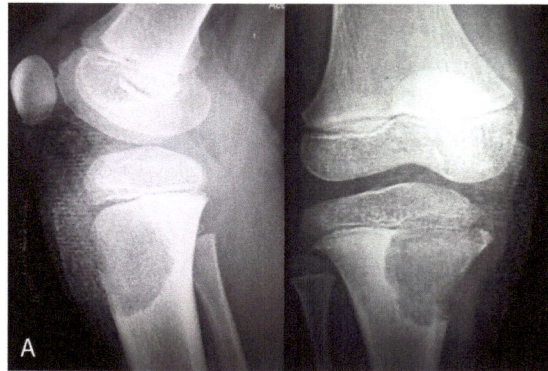

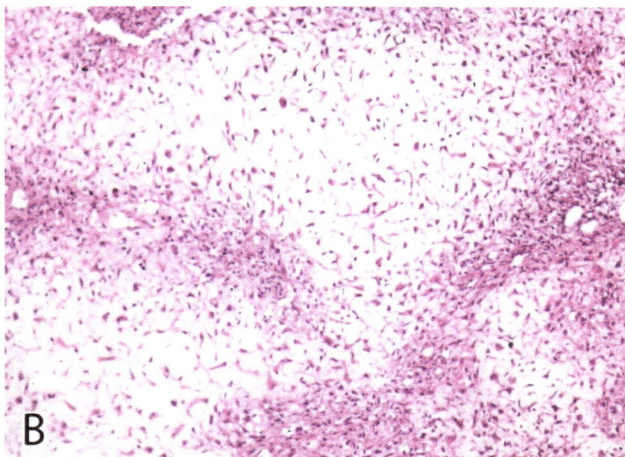

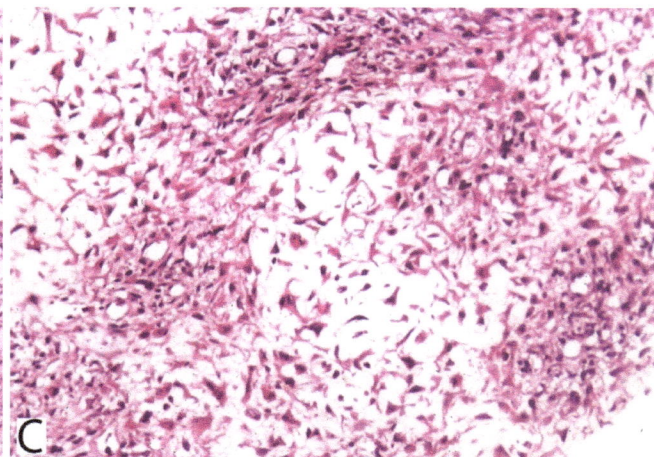

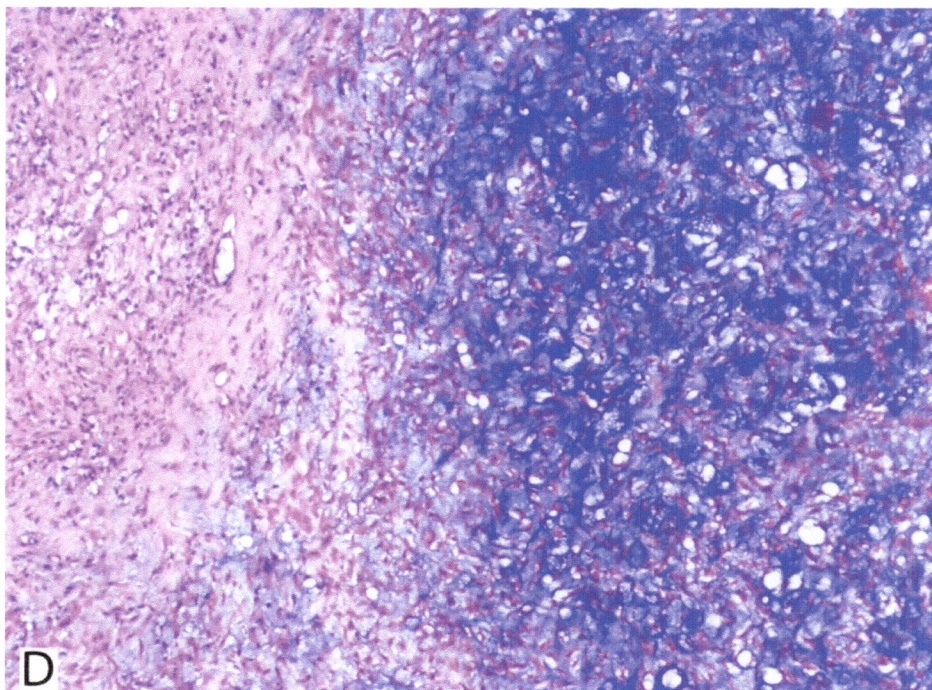

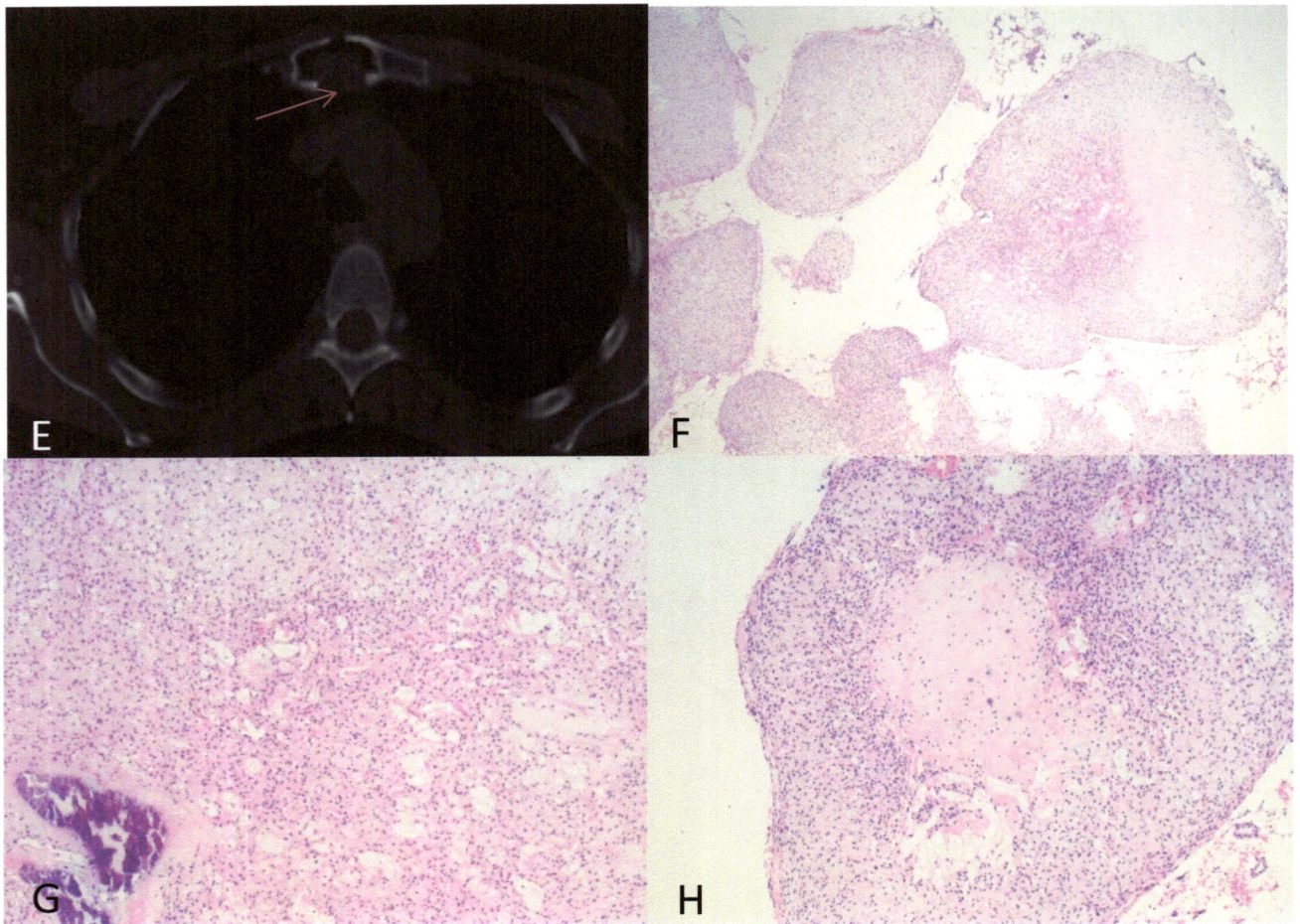

Fig. 2.8 chondromyxoid fibroma: (A) sharply demarcated eccentric osteolytic lesion in metaphysis of upper tibia: lateral and PA view; B&C) well defined islands of spindle and stellate shaped cells in loose sheets, separated by broad septa of compactly arranged neoplastic cells;(D) another case of otherwise typical chondromyxoid fibroma had an occasional island of atypical chondroid tissue; it is difficult to interpret this picture alone without the context.

(E) Chondromyxoid fibroma of manubrium sternum: Fairly demarcated osteolytic lesion in the of manubrium sternum eroding the posterior cortex: CT-scan). (F, G): well circumscribed multinodular mass composed of cytologically bland spindle and stellate cells associated with a focally myxoid and collagenous stroma. (H) Central island of cartilage noted in some areas.

Chondrosarcoma

General considerations

Chondrosarcoma is an incessantly growing destructive tumor of bone that produces cartilaginous matrix but not osteoid. Increased cellularity, nuclear enlargement, atypia and hyperchromasia are not always dependable criteria for diagnosis of chondrosarcoma in short tubular bones, periosteal chondroma and multiple chondromatosis. Destruction of host bone and extension in to the soft tissue are the two most dependable criteria of malignancy in chondroid neoplasms. Chondrosarcoma is slow growing, with bone destruction and soft tissue extension occurring late in the course of the disease. Early diagnosis can be made on the basis of non-histological parameters.

Primary (conventional) chondrosarcoma

Clinical features

Pain is the single most common symptom. It is often described as deep, dull ache that becomes more intense during night. Restriction of movements may occur if the tumor is situated near a major joint. Rarely chondrosarcoma may present with pathologic fracture. Swelling is another common presenting symptom.

Bones of the pelvis, especially ilium, proximal femur, distal femur and ribs are the most commonly affected. Flat bones like pelvis and scapula, long tubular bones (proximal femur, proximal humerus, distal femur) account for 75 % of the cases. . Short tubular bones of the hands and feet which are common sites for enchondromas rarely develop a chondrosarcoma but it behaves as a locally aggressive lesion and, in contrast to chondrosarcomas located elsewhere, rarely metastasizes. Treatment is indicated only because of its locally destructive growth. It is believed that given excellent survival data, curettage with adequate follow-up should be considered as the treatment of choice if technically feasible; especially in those cases in which amputation would lead to a significant loss of hand function[18]. Base of the skull forms another site of chondrosarcoma.

Radiological findings

a) Imaging studies are necessary to establish cartilaginous nature of the tumor; b) to assess destructive nature and possibility of malignancy; and c) to assess extent of the tumor.

The tumor is often located in the metaphysis with fusiform expansion of the shaft (Fig. 9 A). It is lucent with varying degree of mineralization and punctate ring and arc pattern of calcification. This characteristic pattern of mineralization helps in establishing cartilaginous nature of the tumor. When the tumor is predominantly or exclusively lucent, it would be difficult to establish cartilaginous nature. CT scans are more appropriate for demonstrating calcification.

Fusiform expansions of the bone, endosteal erosion / scalloping, cortical thickening are features of malignancy in long tubular bones. Unlike in osteosarcoma, periosteal thickening is not common (Fig. 9 (B). Extension of the tumor in to the soft tissue which is seen better on MRI and is an unequivocal sign of malignancy. Low grade tumors are curetted; these curetted tumors appear greyish blue, translucent, firm. There may be varying degree of myxoid change. Chalky calcification and ossification are common.

Gross

The excised tumor appears lobulated, greyish blue, translucent and firm. Myxoid change and liquefaction are common. Fusiform widening of the bone, cortical thickening and endosteal erosion may be apparent. High grade tumor may appear fleshy with areas of hemorrhage and necrosis. In late stages extension of the tumor in to the soft tissue occurs.

Microscopic

Histological diagnosis of low grade chondrosarcoma requires evidence of bone permeation/ destruction (Fig. 9 C- H). Increased cellularity, and cytological atypia in the proper context i e., in long tubular bones, non-periosteal location and in the absence of multiple chondroma syndromes) are suggestive of malignancy. In high grade tumors nuclear atypia, hyperchromasia are pronounced. Histological diagnosis of high grade chondrosarcomas is easy, and can be made mainly on basis cytological features. Nuclear atypia and hyperchromasia are more pronounced. Necrosis is a feature of high grade tumor. Tumor grade is the most important parameter that helps in therapeutic decision making and in prognostication. Grading is done on scale of 1 to 3 based on cellularity, nuclear atypia and hyperchromasia. Majority (61%) of chondrosarcomas are grade I tumors; 36 % are grade II ; while only 3% are grade III tumor. Grade 1 tumors resemble enchondroma to a great extent. In limited biopsy material non-histological parameters are necessary to buttress the diagnosis of malignancy. There may be mild to moderate increase in cellularity with occasional enlarged nuclei and mild to moderate hyperchromasia. More than occasional binucleate cells are seen. Mitosis is indeed rare (Fig. 9 C, D, E, F, G, and H)

Grade 2 tumors are more cellular than grade 1 tumors with easily identifiable enlarged and hyperchromatic nuclei (Fig. 10 A, B, C, D). There are more easily identifiable binucleate cells. Mitosis is still rare.

Grade 3 tumors are distinctly cellular with far more nuclear anaplasia than in grade 2 tumors. There may be necrosis. Mitosis is seen (Fig. 11A, B).

High grade chondrosarcoma in adolescents and young should raise the possibility of conventional high grade osteosarcoma even in the absence of osteoid.

Grade 1 sarcomas in long tubular bones are curetted; while for grade 2 and grade 3 tumors, en-block resection is advised.

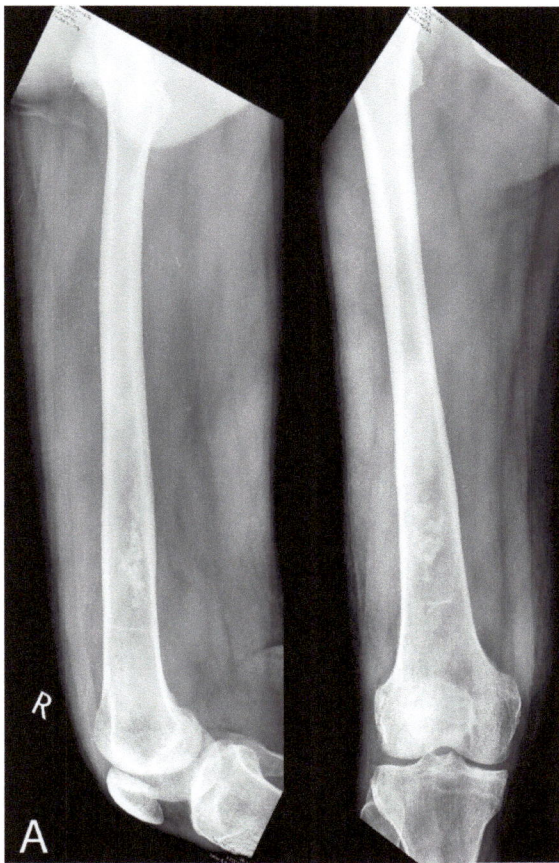

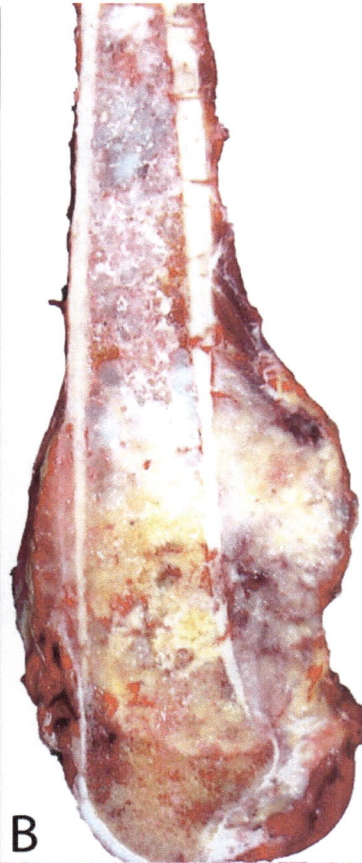

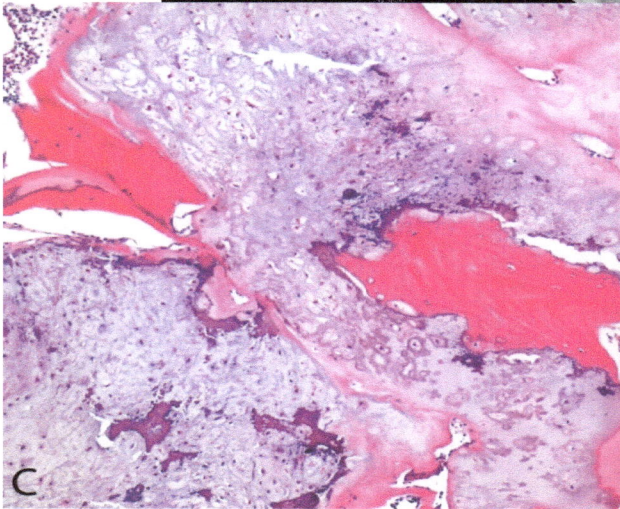

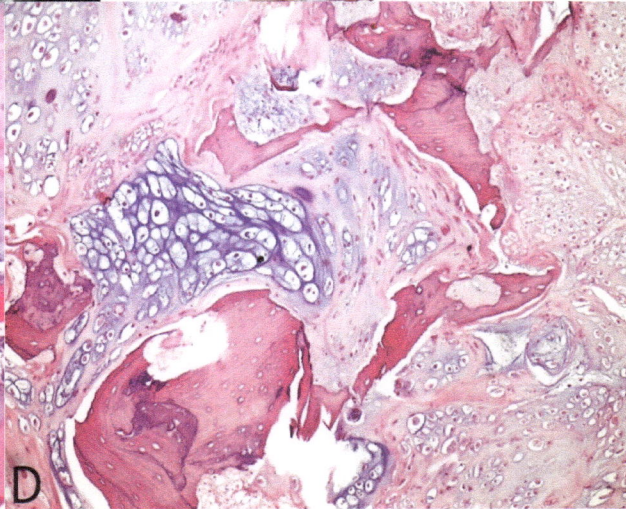

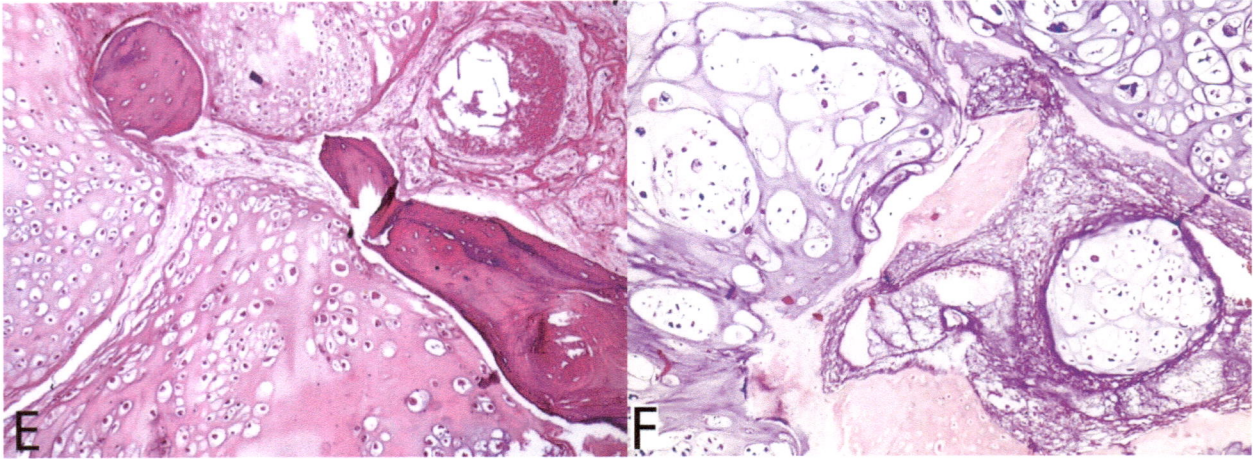

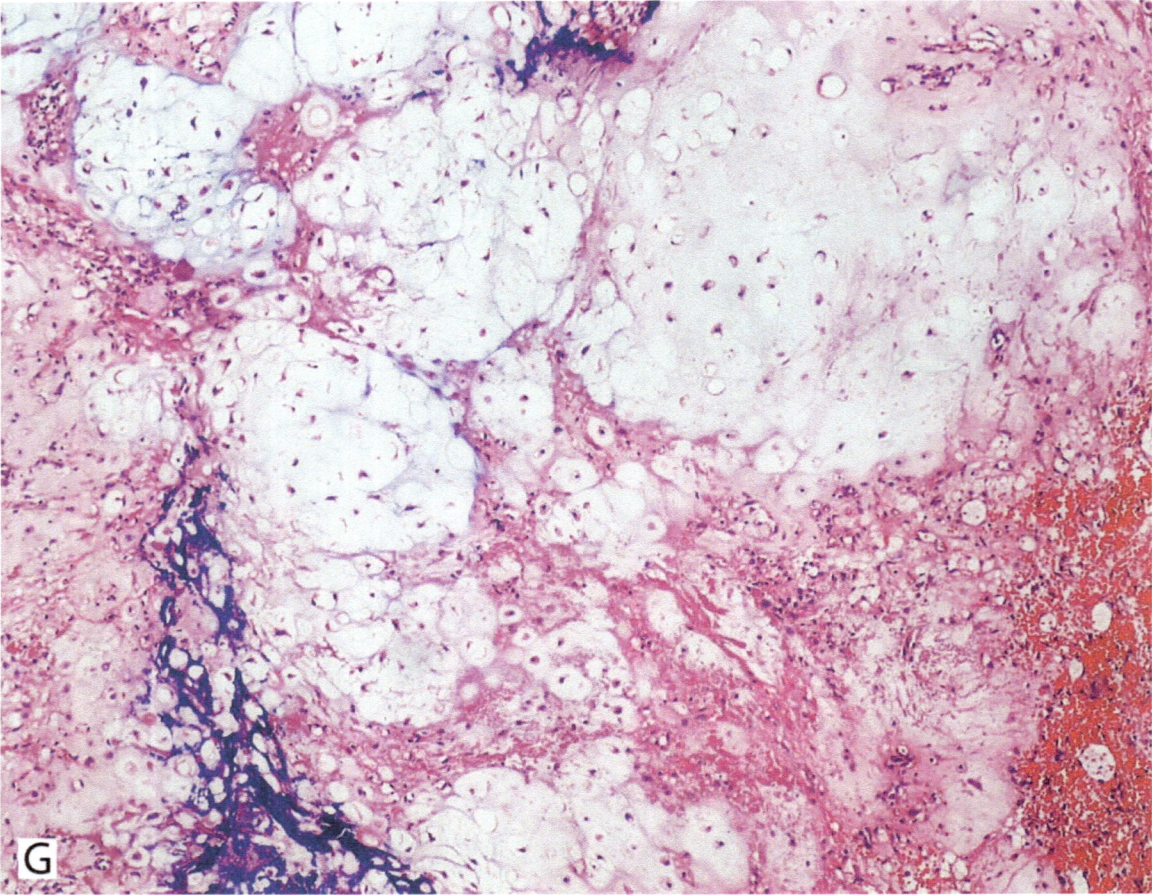

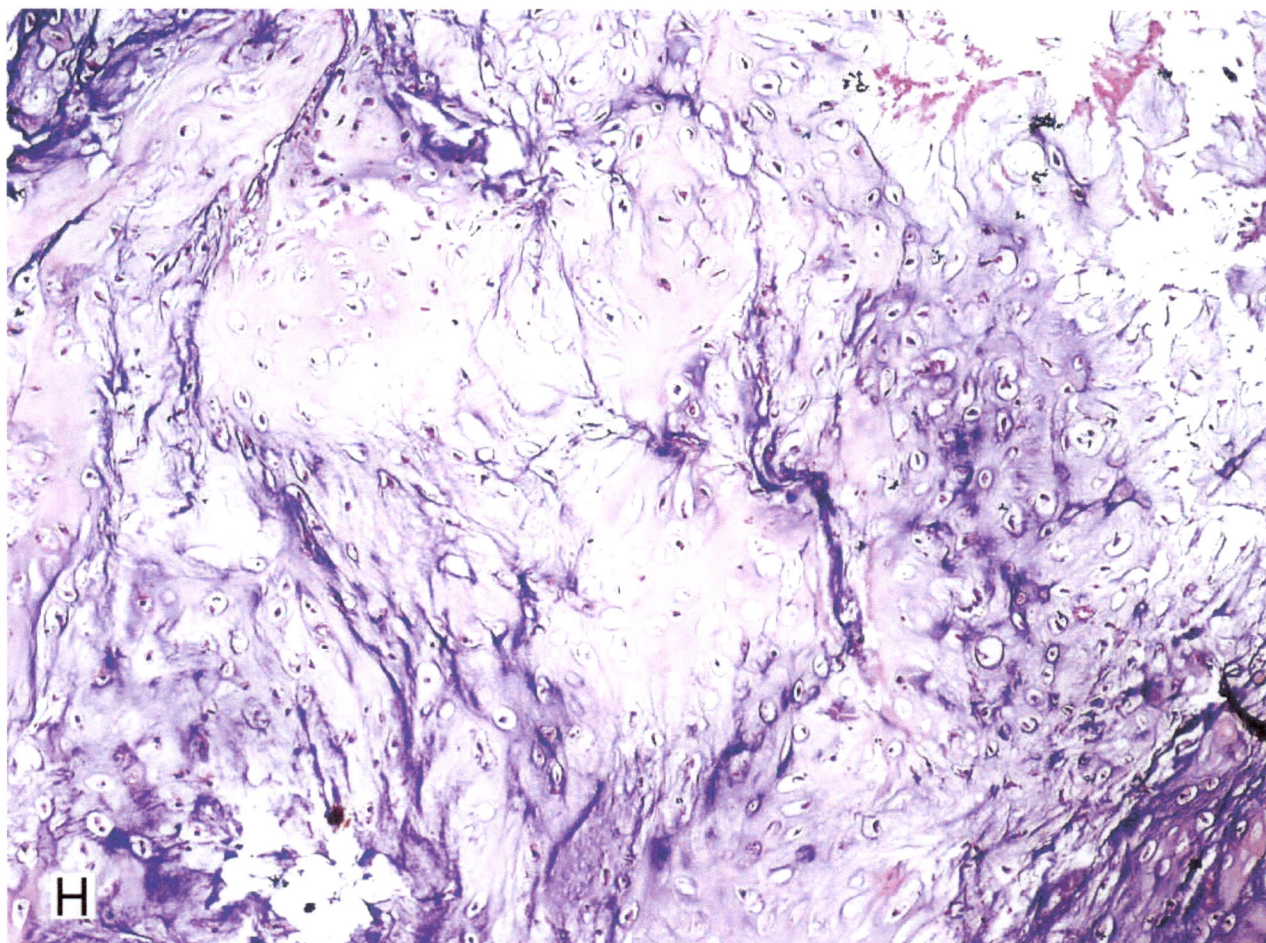

Fig. 2.9 Primary chondrosarcoma: (A) lesion in lower half of femur with rings and arcs calcification, and suspicious cortical erosion; (B) medullary cavity containing yellowish brown and bluish cartilage islands, with extensive soft tissue involvement; C,D,E,F,G,H) grade 1 chondrosarcoma with destruction of the bone.

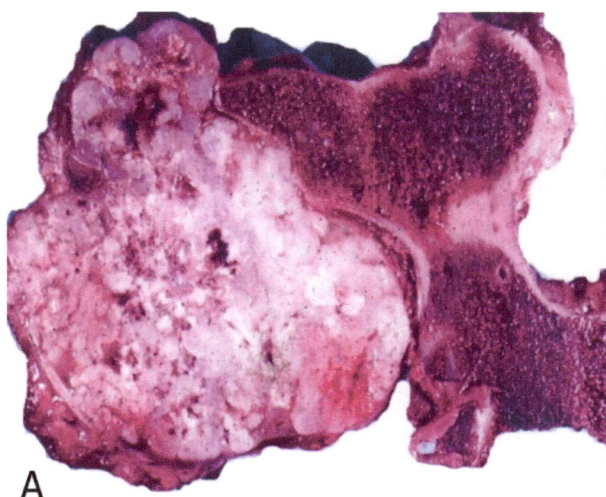

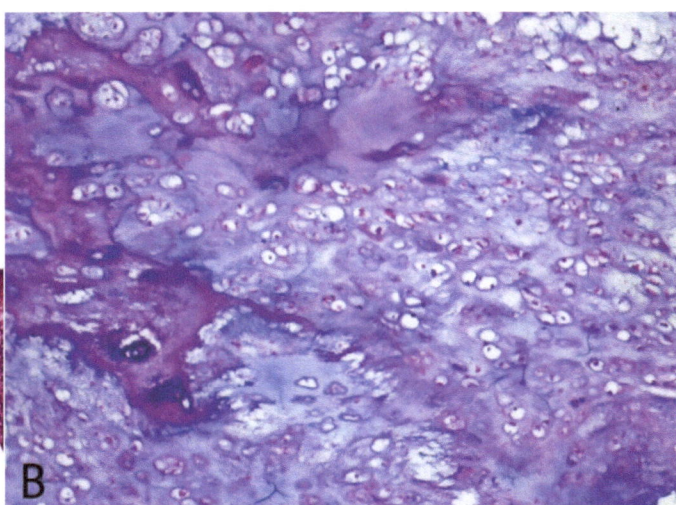

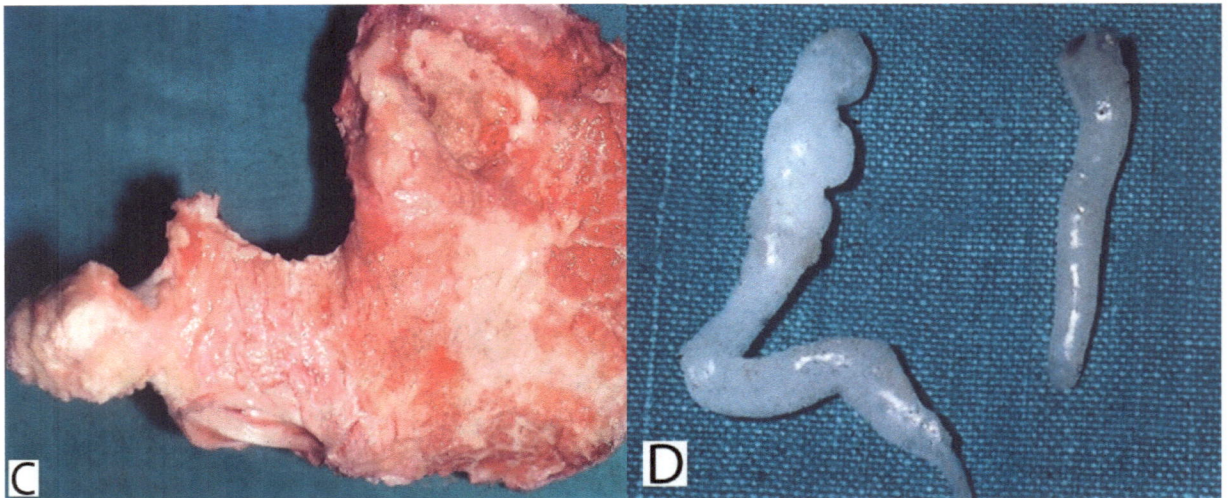

Fig. 2.10 primary chondrosarcomas: (A) well defined bulky chondroid neoplasm of pelvis; (B) histologically, grade II chondrosarcoma; (C) diffusely involved iliac bone with grade II whitish tumor; (D) cartilaginous tumor emboli from surrounding major pelvic veins (same case as C)

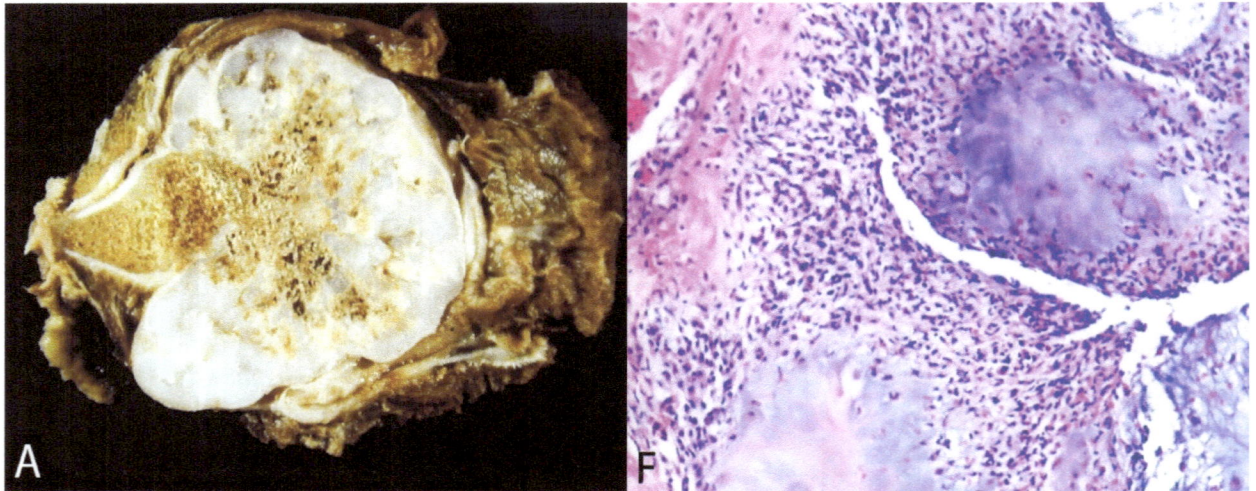

Fig. 2.11 (A) large, lobulated circumscribed glistening white tumor of pelvis; (B) histologically, grade III chondrosarcoma (the same case as in A)

Prognosis

For chondrosarcoma the prognosis depends mainly on grade of the tumor. Grade 1 tumors are locally aggressive, and may recur; metastasis is exceptional. Recurrent tumor may show higher grade. The five-year survival rate for grade 1 tumors is estimated to be 83 % ; and for grade 2 and 3 tumors, 53 %. Overall survival rates for patients with localized chondrosarcoma in a series of 115 patients was 79% and 69% respectively for five years and 10 year follow up[19]. The event-free survival was significantly better for patients with chondrosarcoma of extremities than those of patients with chondrosarcoma of axial skeleton and pelvic girdle[19]. The biological evolution of chondrosarcoma is slow, requiring long follow up intervals for meaningful survival analysis. A study of 344 patients (M:F 1.3:1.0) of primary chondrosarcoma over a period of 80 years, revealed that with adequate initial surgical intervention chondrosarcoma is primarily a local disease with low metastatic rate[20].

Secondary peripheral chondrosarcoma

Chondrosarcoma arising in a pre-existing osteochondroma is called secondary peripheral chondrosarcoma (Fig. 12 A, B,C). The incidence is estimated to be 1% in solitary osteochondromas, while it is higher (5%) in multiple osteochondromas. Secondary chondrosarcomas occur at younger age compared to primary chondrosarcomas. In a study of 107 secondary chondrosarcomas, 61 patients had solitary osteochondroma, and 46 had multiple osteochondromas. 5- and 10-year mortality rate was 1.6% and 4.8% respectively. Five patients died of metastatic disease and others of local recurrences only [21].

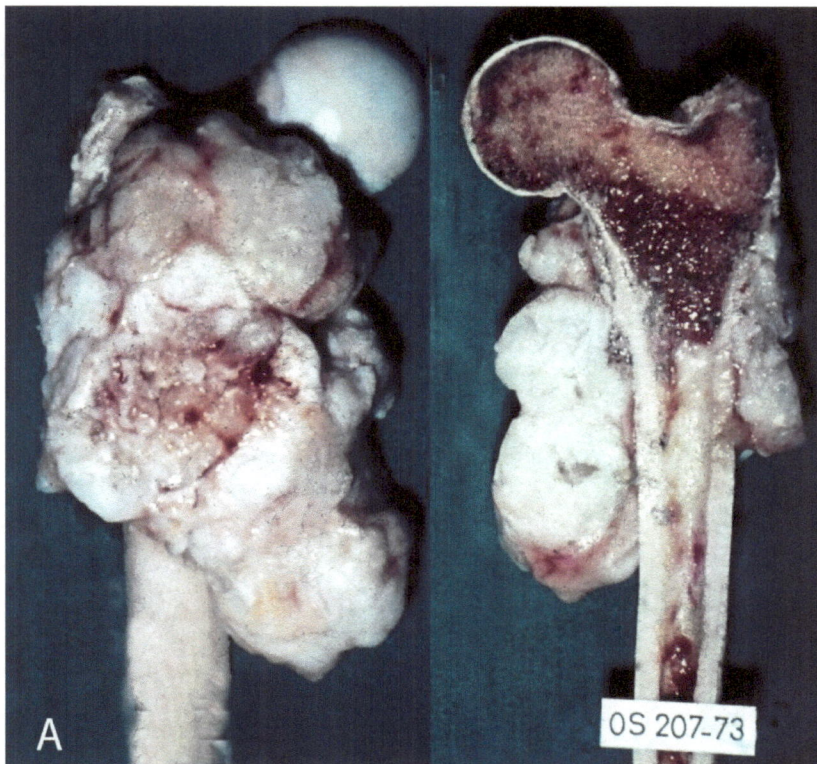

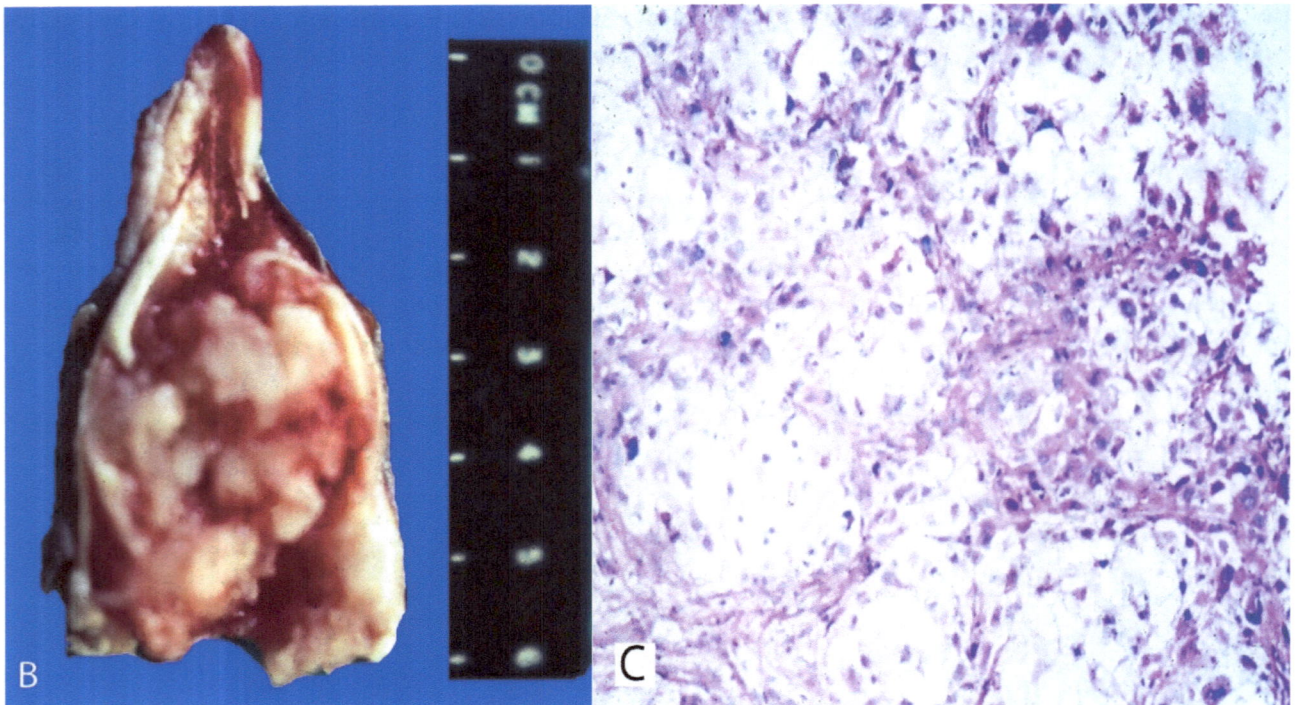

Fig. 2.12 Secondary chondrosarcoma: (A) large histologically well differentiated chondrosarcoma arising from an osteochondroma, diagnosed as osteochondroma on x-ray 14 years ago and left untreated; (B) a case of enchondroma curetted at the age of 29 years, recurred 11 years later; (C) this particular secondary chondrosarcoma is high grade (grade III), although secondary chondrosarcomas are usually of low grade malignancy

Clinically, development of pain, rapid increase in size or pathologic fracture at the site of a known osteochondroma should lead to suspicion of secondary chondrosarcoma.

In a Mayo clinic series of 75 cases of chondrosarcomas secondary to osteochondroma, 40 patients had single exostosis and 35 had multiple lesions. More males than females were affected, and most of the patients were age 20 to 40 years. The tumors involved various bones. Malignant change was manifested radiologically by fuzzy margins of the cartilage cap and by the presence of lucent zones within the lesion. Grossly, the surface of the thickened cartilage cap was irregular. Microscopically, most of the tumors were well-differentiated (Grade 1). Treatment was surgical. Simple excision of the tumor resulted in a large recurrence rate. En block resection and amputation were generally curative [22].

Bone sarcomas associated with multiple enchondromatosis syndrome

About 25 % of Ollier's disease patients develop secondary chondrosarcomas. This incidence is 15 % in patients who have involvement of the short bones of hands and feet and is about 40 % in whom long bone are also involved [23]. Incidence in Maffucci syndrome is much higher (53 %) (Fig. 13 A, B, C, D).

Gross and histological features of malignancy in these cases are the same as in conventional chondrosarcomas with one caveat that in tumors associated with Ollier's disease and Maffucci syndrome, chondromas do show alarming features like increased cellularity and mild to moderate nuclear atypia and hyperchromasia. Hence, in these cases diagnosis of malignancy cannot be made solely on the basis of cytological features. Additional features of aggressiveness like permeation, and entrapment of the host bone, disruption of the cortex, and extension of tumor in to the soft tissue should be looked for.

Of 55 patients with Ollier's disease seen at the Mayo Clinic between 1907 and 1985, 16 had malignant bone neoplasms: 12 chondrosarcomas, two dedifferentiated chondrosarcomas, one chordoma, and one osteosarcoma. These findings suggest that approximately 30% of patients with Ollier's disease will develop a malignant bone neoplasm, most probably chondrosarcoma. The prognosis for most patients is good. Five of the 16 patients survived more than 13 years after treatment [24].

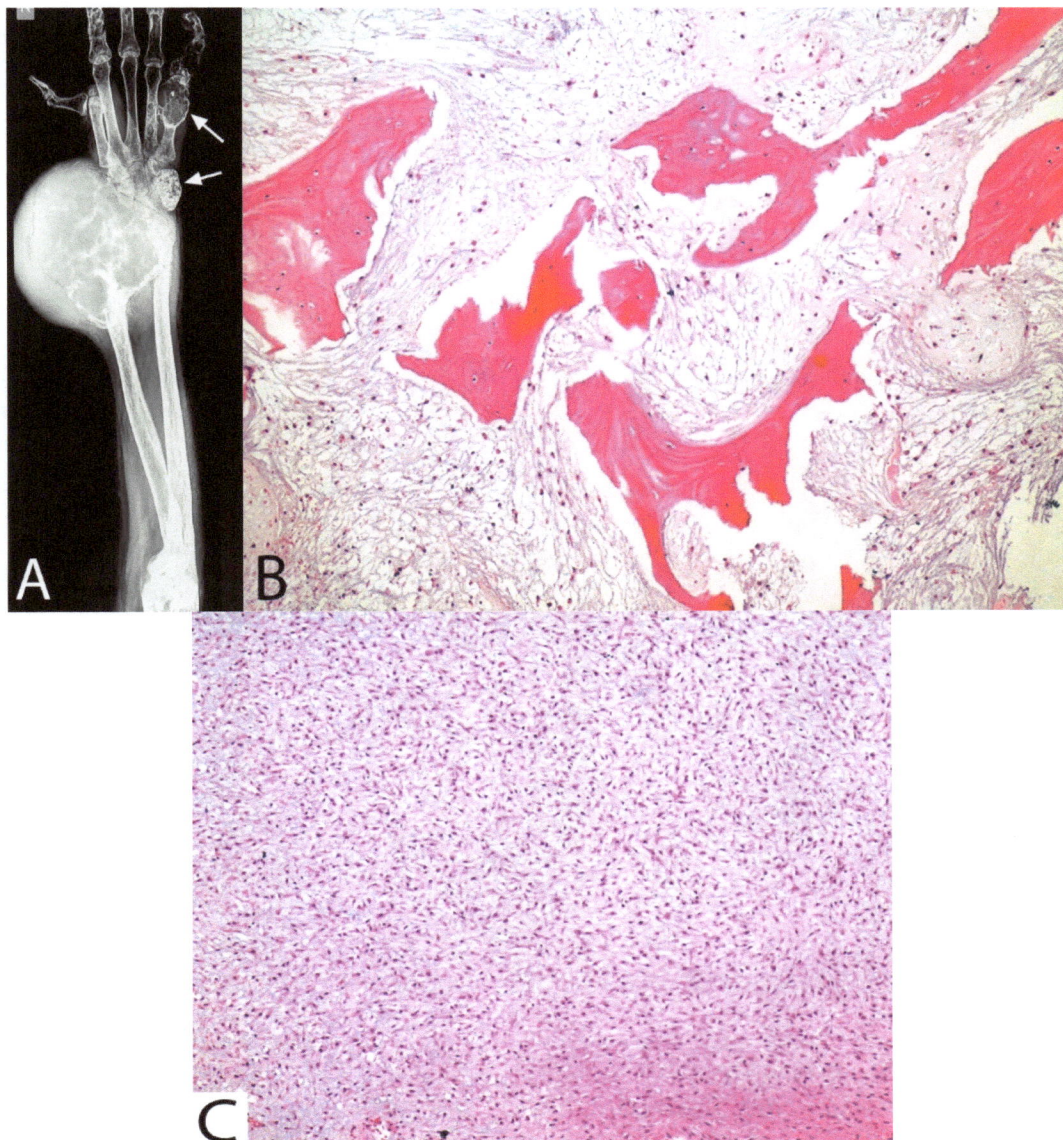

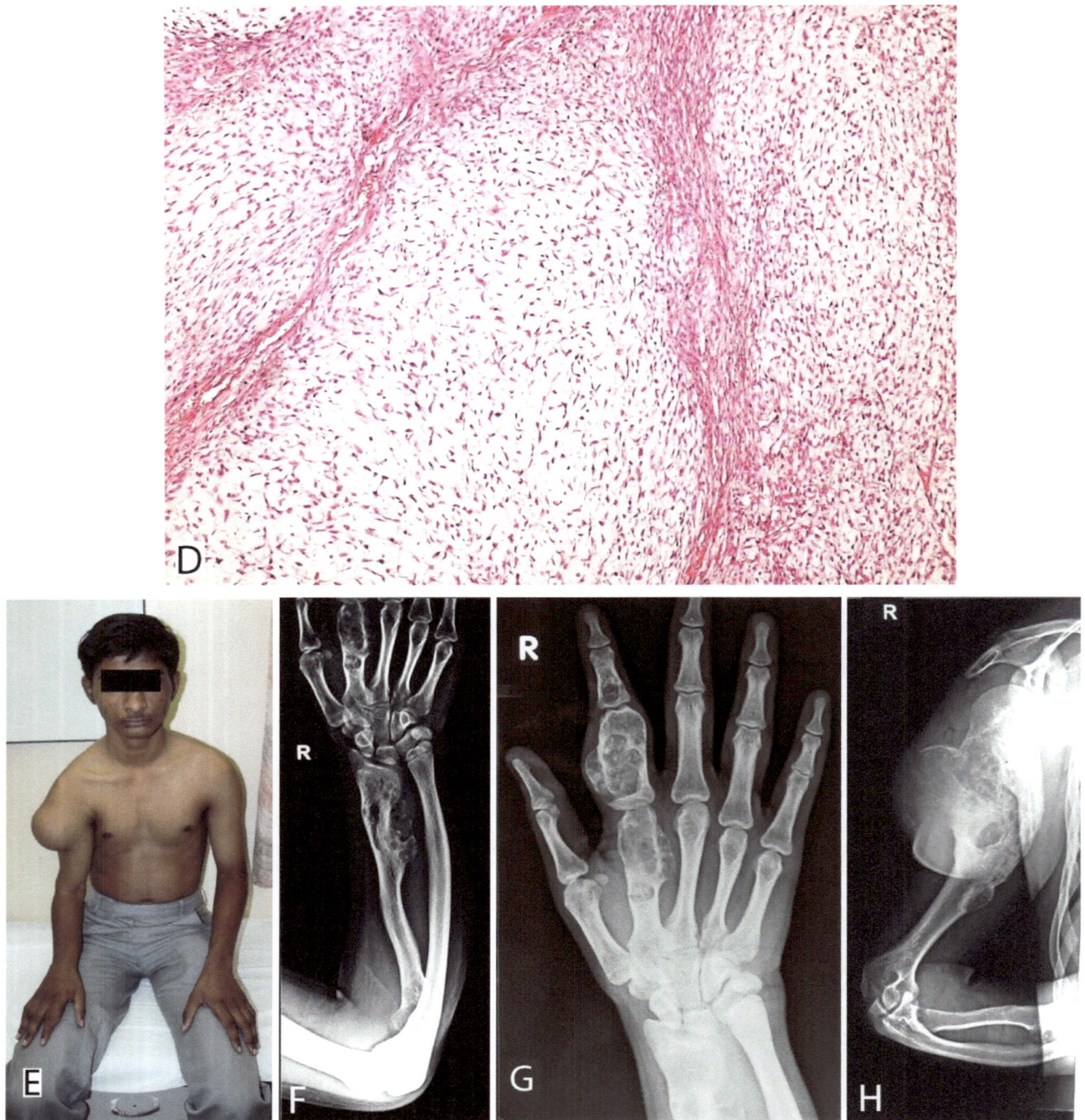

Fig. 2.13 (A) Secondary chondrosarcoma of proximal radius in a case of Maffucci's syndrome, note enchondromas in the hand bones (arrows), this patient also had soft tissue angiomatosis in the foot; (B &C) chondrosarcoma grade 2 from this case: moderately cellular small cell chondroid population with intercellular basophilic mucoid matrix (D) chondrosarcoma grade II from a different case of secondary chondrosarcoma, the myxoid pattern is characteristic; (E) Another case of Ollier's disease showing large smooth oval tumor mass arising from upper humerus; (F) enchondromas in small bones of hand and chondrosarcoma arising from lower end of radius with extension in soft tissues; (G)three enchondromas in small bones of hand and chondrosarcoma in the distal radius; (H) large destructive chondrosarcoma involving epi-metaphysis and upper diaphysis of humerus, the same tumor shown in clinical picture E.

Dedifferentiated chondrosarcoma

The concept of dedifferentiated chondrosarcomas was put forth by Dahlin and Beabout[25] in 1971 Juxtaposition of low grade chondrosarcoma adjacent to high grade heterologous non-cartilaginous sarcoma was interpreted as 'dedifferentiation'. This concept of 'dedifferentiation' is now extended to non-cartilaginous tumors including epithelial tumors. About 11% of low grade chondrosarcomas undergo dedifferentiation. The sarcomatous component is usually osteosarcoma, undifferentiated high grade pleomorphic sarcoma (Malignant fibrous histiocytoma); fibrosarcoma and rarely rhabdomyosarcoma type [26] and behaves very aggressively (Fig. 14 B, C).

Radiologically [27], the dedifferentiated chondrosarcoma is like any chondrosarcoma with additional features of lucent areas with cortical destruction (Fig. 14 A). The lucent areas represent the high grade non-cartilaginous sarcoma component. MRI and PET scan would effectively delineate the two components in most cases. The ability to predict the possibility of dedifferentiation in a low-grade chondrosarcoma on the basis of imaging is critical to ensure adequate sampling at the time of biopsy.

Prognosis

Grimer et al [28] reported a data on 337 patients of dedifferentiated chondrosarcoma from nine European centers: 71 patients (21%) had metastases at the time of diagnosis and had a 10% chance of survival at 2 years. The prognosis for patients with this tumor remains dismal and surgery with clear margins remains the principle treatment.

Metastatic disease at diagnosis, Undifferentiated high grade pleomorphic sarcoma (Malignant fibrous histiocytoma) dedifferentiation, and a high percentage of dedifferentiated components are related to poorer outcomes. There was no statistical evidence of any beneficial effect from adjuvant chemotherapy [29].

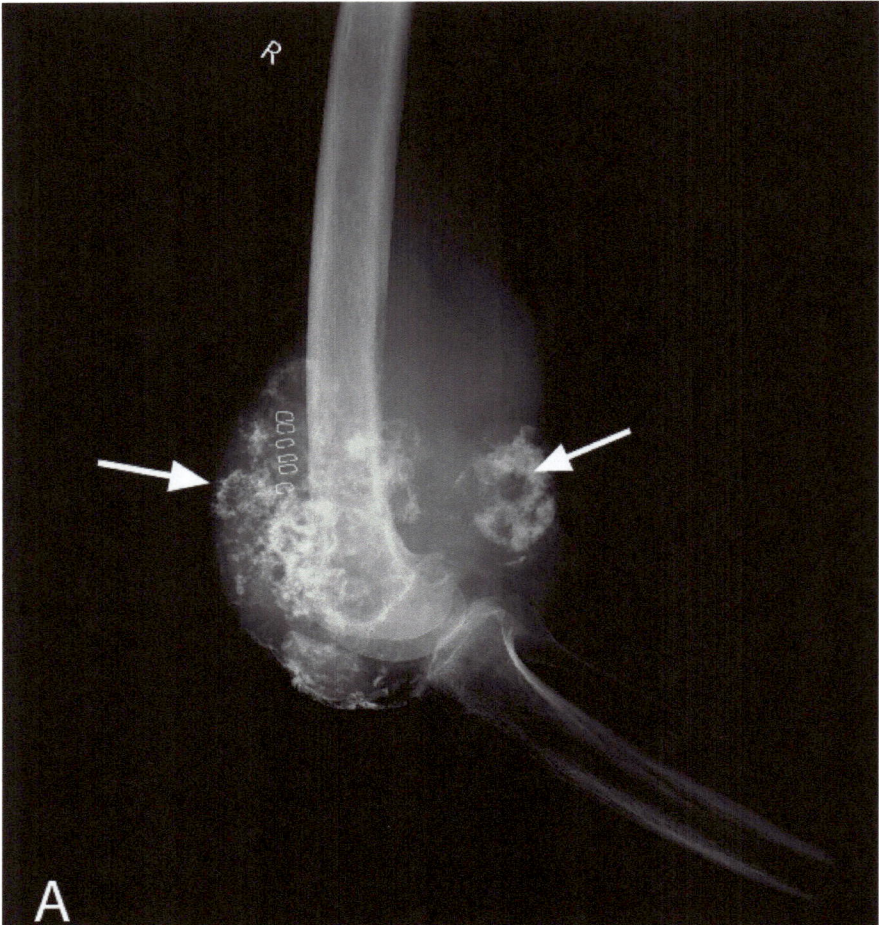

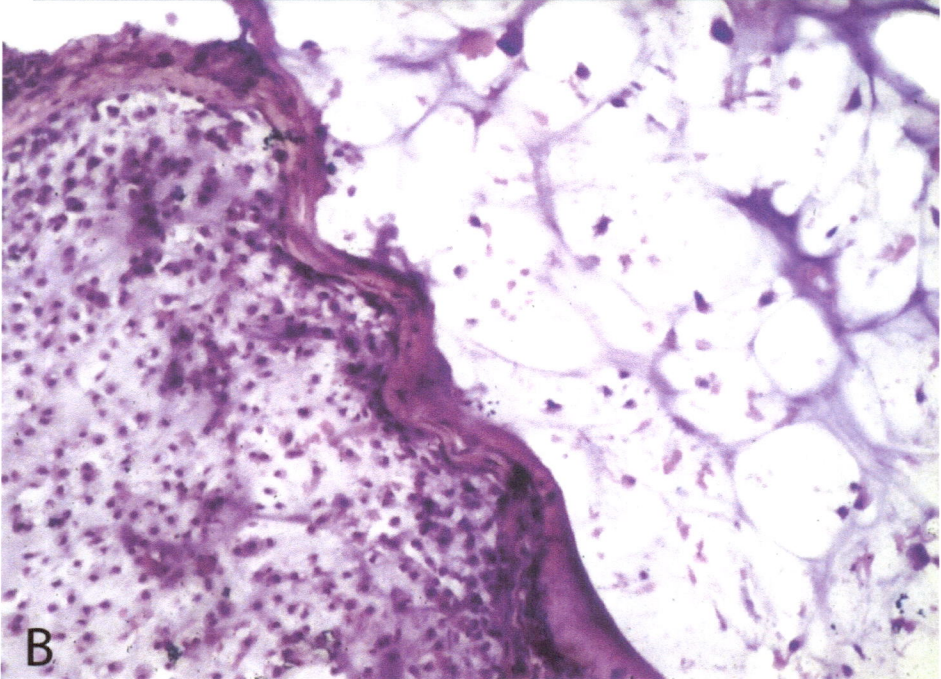

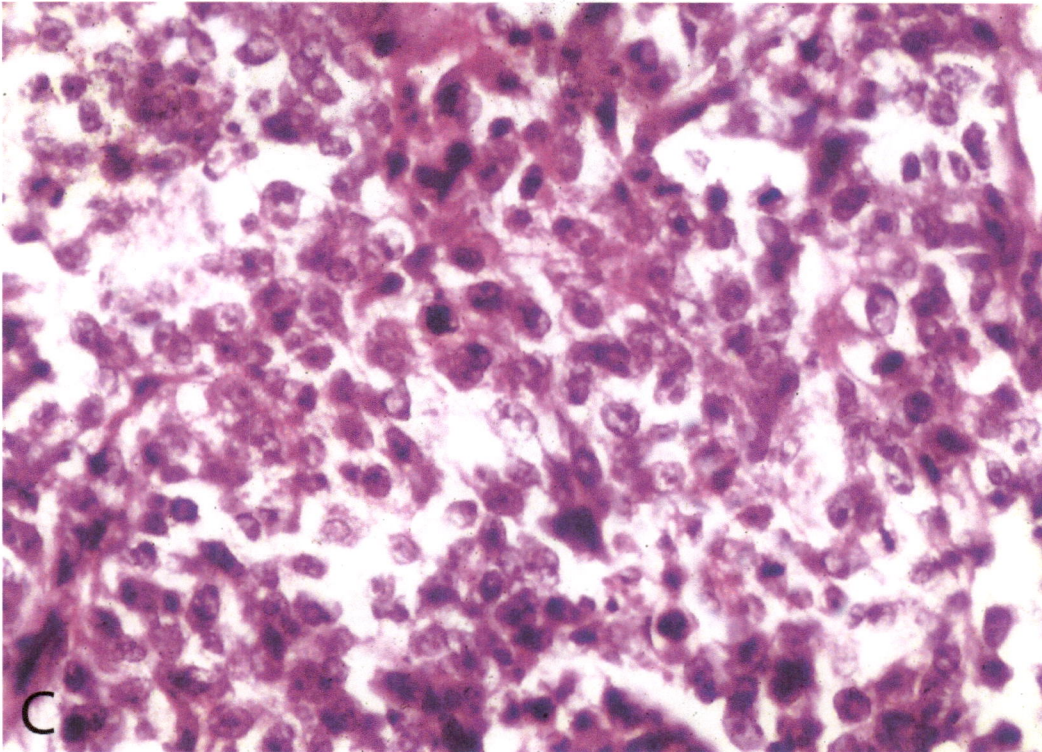

Fig. 2.14 Dedifferentiated chondrosarcoma: (A) X ray of the knee joint lateral view showing cartilaginous tumor with lytic areas (arrows) indicating soft cellular dedifferentiated component; (B) in a known case of grade 1 chondrosarcoma, is seen an area of grade III chondrosarcoma; (C) at second recurrence in the same case, undifferentiated mesenchymal tumor was identified.

Clear cell chondrosarcoma

Clear cell chondrosarcoma is a rare distinct low grade malignant tumor, which presents diagnostic difficulties. Its clinical, radiological, and morphologic characteristics separate it from conventional chondrosarcoma and some benign bone tumors with which it is often confused. In a series of 47 cases from Mayo Clinic [30] age of occurrence was in 3rd and 4th decades. The tumor has distinct predilection for males with male: female ratio of 2.6:1. The lesions tend to involve ends of long bones, particularly upper end of humerus and upper end of femur, similar to chondroblastoma and giant cell tumors. The radiographic appearance (Fig.15 A) may mimic that of chondroblastoma in that the lesion is usually well circumscribed and may even have sclerotic border [31].

It is characterized histologically by sheets of clear cells, resembling chondrocytes, islands of hyaline cartilage, scattered fragments of woven bone and multinucleated osteoclastic giant cells. The tumor cells have well-defined cytoplasmic borders and a centrally placed nucleus often containing a nucleolus (Fig. 15 B, C, D). In some cases, foci of conventional chondrosarcoma are detected [32].

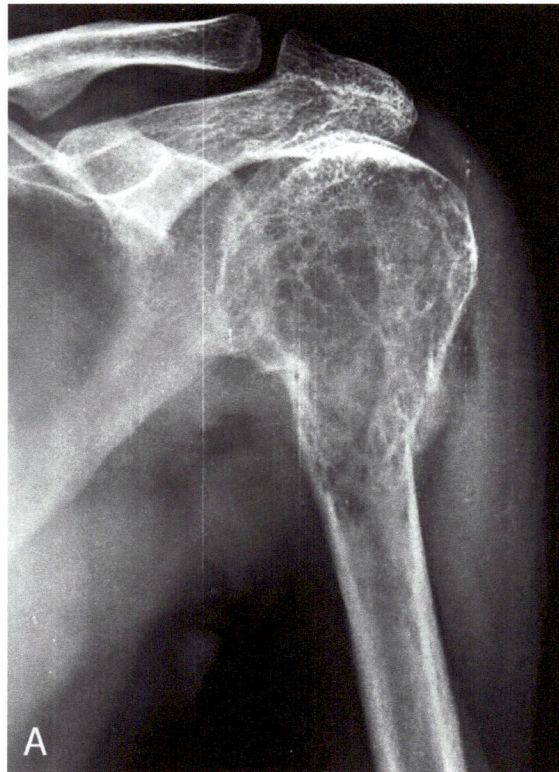

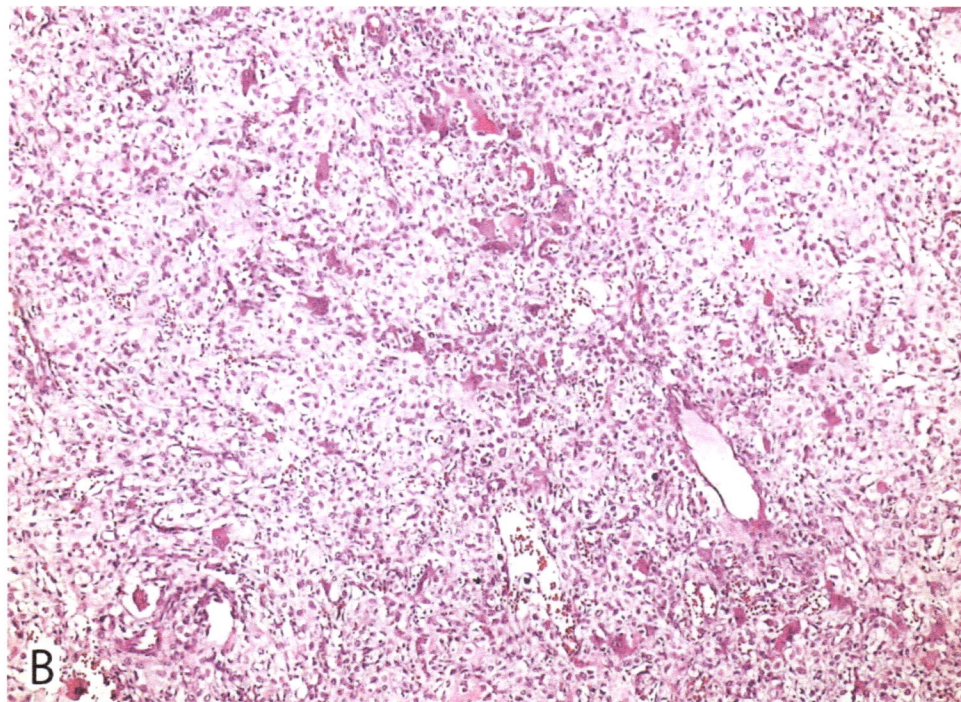

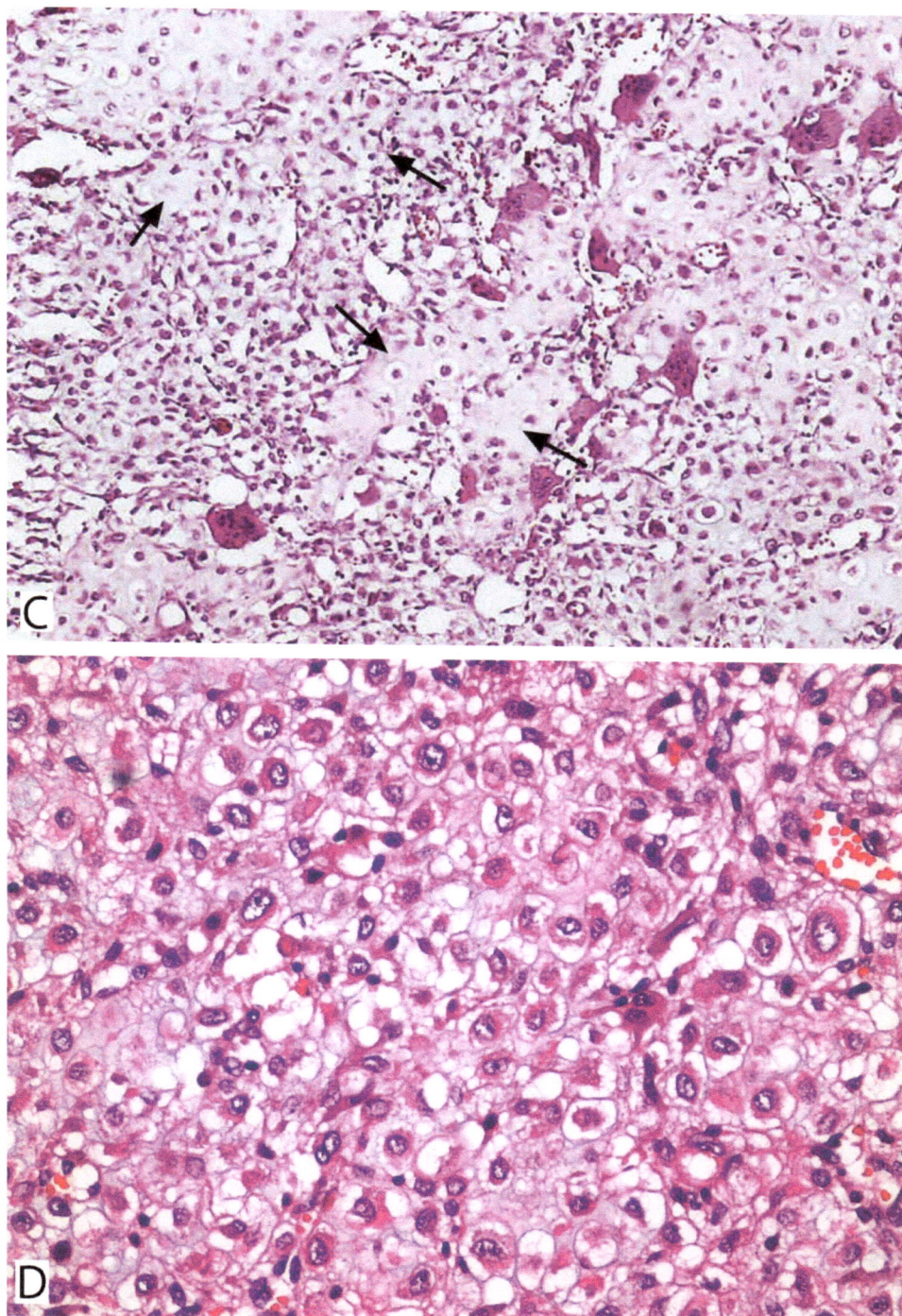

Fig.2.15 Clear cell chondrosarcoma: (A) X-ray shows expanded humeral epiphysis with large lucent lesion, not unlike that of conventional giant cell tumor ; (B) at low power, sheets of clear cells, osteoclastic giant cells and minimal bone formation are seen; (C) large rounded cells with clear cytoplasm and well defined cell borders, evenly spread osteoclastic cells, and islands of hyaline cartilage (arrows) area seen, note some resemblance to chondroblastoma; (D) cells with clear and eosinophilic cytoplasm like in chondroblasts.

Prognosis

Clear cell chondrosarcoma has a slowly progressive clinical course and infrequent metastasis, but with a high local recurrence rate. Of the 16 patients with this tumor who had long-term clinical follow-up, three had local recurrence, and four developed metastatic disease with a median time of 8.1 years after diagnosis. Ten-year overall survival was 89% and disease free survival was 68%, in one series [33].

Mesenchymal chondrosarcoma

Mesenchymal chondrosarcoma is a rare high grade biphasic sarcoma composed of undifferentiated small round cells and islands of well differentiated hyaline cartilage. It occurs within bones and less commonly soft tissues. In a review of 111 cases [34], the age range was 5 to 74 years with approximately 60% of cases reported in the second and third decades of life. Seventy-two tumors arose in bone and 38 were found in extra skeletal sites. In another series of 20 cases of mesenchymal chondrosarcoma the anatomical sites are quite widespread: eighteen tumors (90%) originated in bone, and 2 tumors (10%) were of extraskeletal origin; of the skeletal tumors, locations included craniofacial bones (n = 9; 50%), ribs and chest wall (n = 4; 22%), sacrum and spinal elements (n = 3; 17%), and lower extremities (n = 2; 11%), whereas soft tissue tumors were located about the scapula (n = 1; 50%) and lower extremity (n = 1; 50%) [35]. Meningeal involvement has also been reported.

Radiologically, the lesions in bone frequently resemble conventional chondrosarcomas, showing osteolytic and destructive appearance with stippled calcification. Tumors in extra skeletal sites are almost always identified as calcified masses (Fig. 16 A).

Gross

The tumor is greyish white, soft to firm with cartilaginous nodules (Fig. 16 B).

Microscopic

Histologically this is a biphasic tumor composed of high grade small round cell component with necrosis, and islands of hyaline cartilage. Proportion of small round cell component and hyaline cartilage component varies from case to case, and area to area. The small round cell component on its own may easily be mistaken for Ewing sarcoma or any other type of small round cell malignant tumor (Fig. 16 C, D), particularly in needle biopsy specimens. Hemangiopericytoma-like pattern (Fig. 16 E), characterized by solid cellular islands and sheets of small tumor cells separated by elongated vascular spaces, has been frequently encountered in mesenchymal chondrosarcoma. A potential overlap with Ewing sarcoma is enhanced by the fact that more than 90% of mesenchymal chondrosarcomas show strong diffuse membranous immunoreactivity for CD99. However, FLI-1 is positive in 75% of Ewing sarcoma and negative in mesenchymal chondrosarcoma [36].

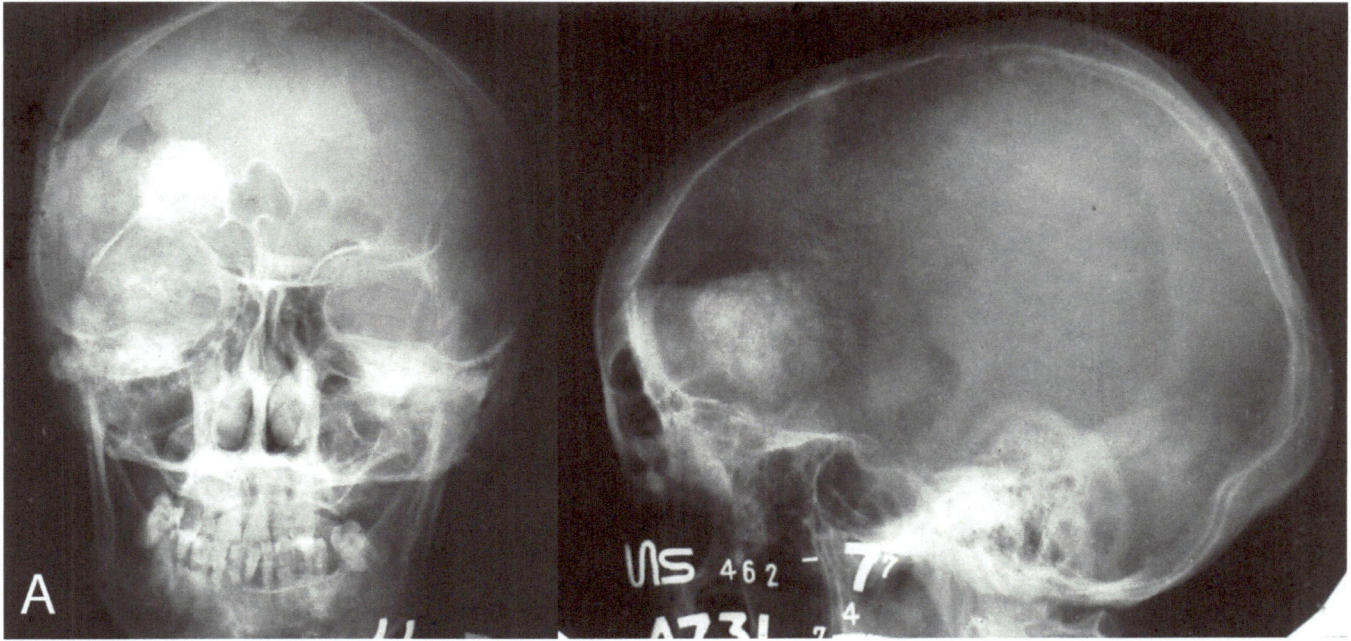

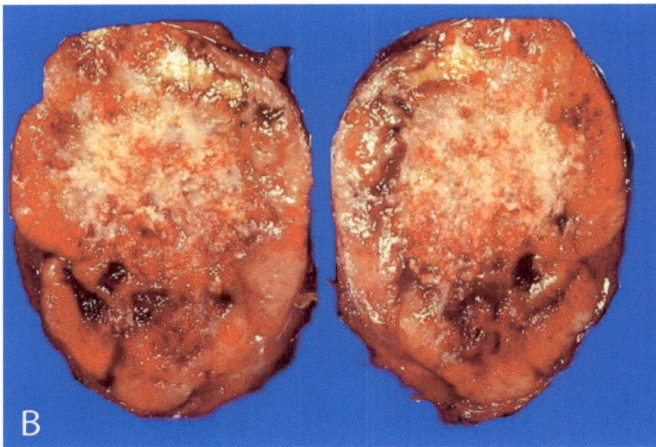

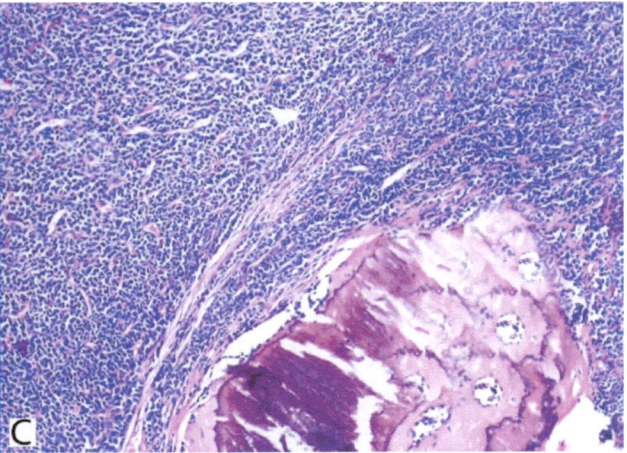

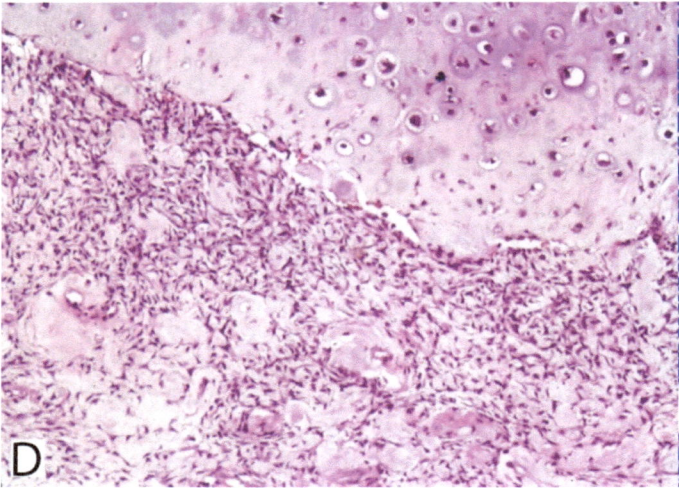

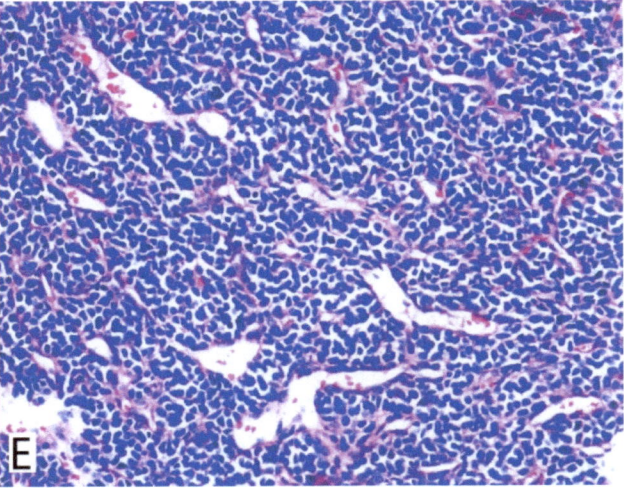

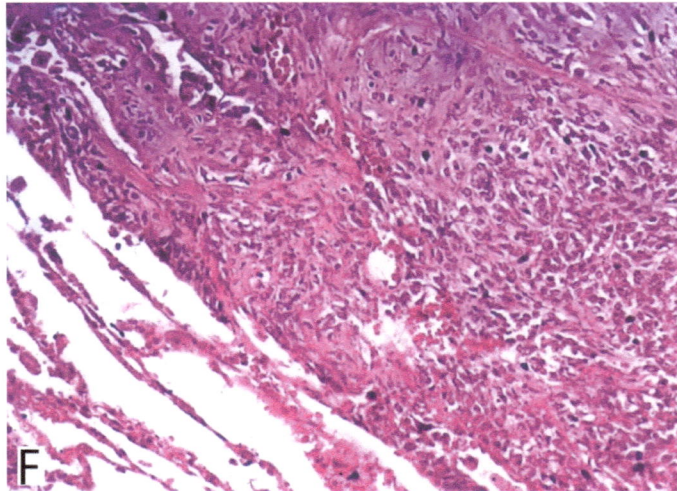

Fig. 2.16: mesenchymal chondrosarcoma: (A) lateral and AP plain x-ray view of a circumscribed calcified lesion in the frontal region; (B) the excised oval tumor shows a large central area of calcification, (C) solid cellular small cell malignant tumor with nodule of differentiated cartilage; (D) a chondroid nodule in upper half; (E) hemangiopericytomatous pattern; (F) metastasis of mesenchymal chondrosarcoma in lung

Prognosis

Although, there are many case reports and case series, the tumor is poorly understood, particularly from the point of optimal management. The consistently described features of mesenchymal chondrosarcoma are unique: biphasic histology and high incidence of metastatic disease (Fig. 16 (F)).

The prognosis of mesenchymal chondrosarcoma is usually poor, and long term follow-up is necessary. Mesenchymal chondrosarcoma is a rare, almost uniformly lethal variant of chondrosarcoma which has been regarded as resistant to chemotherapy and radiotherapy. Seventeen cases are reported; 14 are dead of tumor or still alive with disease; eight of the 14 died less than one year after treatment, predominately of distant metastatic disease [37].

Skeletal Myxoid chondrosarcoma ("Chordoid" sarcoma)

Enzinger and Shiraki (1972) [38] described a rare entity called extraskeletal myxoid chondrosarcoma in a series of 34 tumors occurring in deep muscles of extremities. The tumor consisted of nodular masses of cords and strands of small acidophilic cells, separated by abundant myxoid matrix. Cartilaginous origin of cells was suggested by close resemblance to developing chondroblasts, histochemical features of the matrix, and ultrastructural findings. Many cases of extraskeletal myxoid chondrosarcoma have been published in the literature but true skeletal myxoid chondrosarcoma has been seldom reported. The case illustrated here shows multiloculated destructive tumor in the calcaneum. The gross reveals nodules of predominantly myxoid tumor (Fig. 17 A, B).

Extraskeletal and skeletal myxoid chondrosarcomas histologically appear identical (Fig. 18 A, B) and were considered to be the same tumor with a common histogenesis. However, fundamental differences have been noted at the ultrastructural and molecular levels, suggesting that these tumors represent two distinct entities in the chondrosarcoma family. Antonescu et al made a comparative clinicopathologic and molecular study with 20 cases of extraskeletal and 20 cases of skeletal myxoid chondrosarcoma. Histologically, all cases revealed 95% myxoid matrix with only minimal (5%) cartilage formation. Cytogenetic evaluation demonstrated the presence of recurrent translocation t (9; 22) (q 22-31; q11-12) in extraskeletal tumors. This is the molecular signature pathognomonic of extraskeletal myxoid chondrosarcoma and has not been found in other mesenchymal tumors

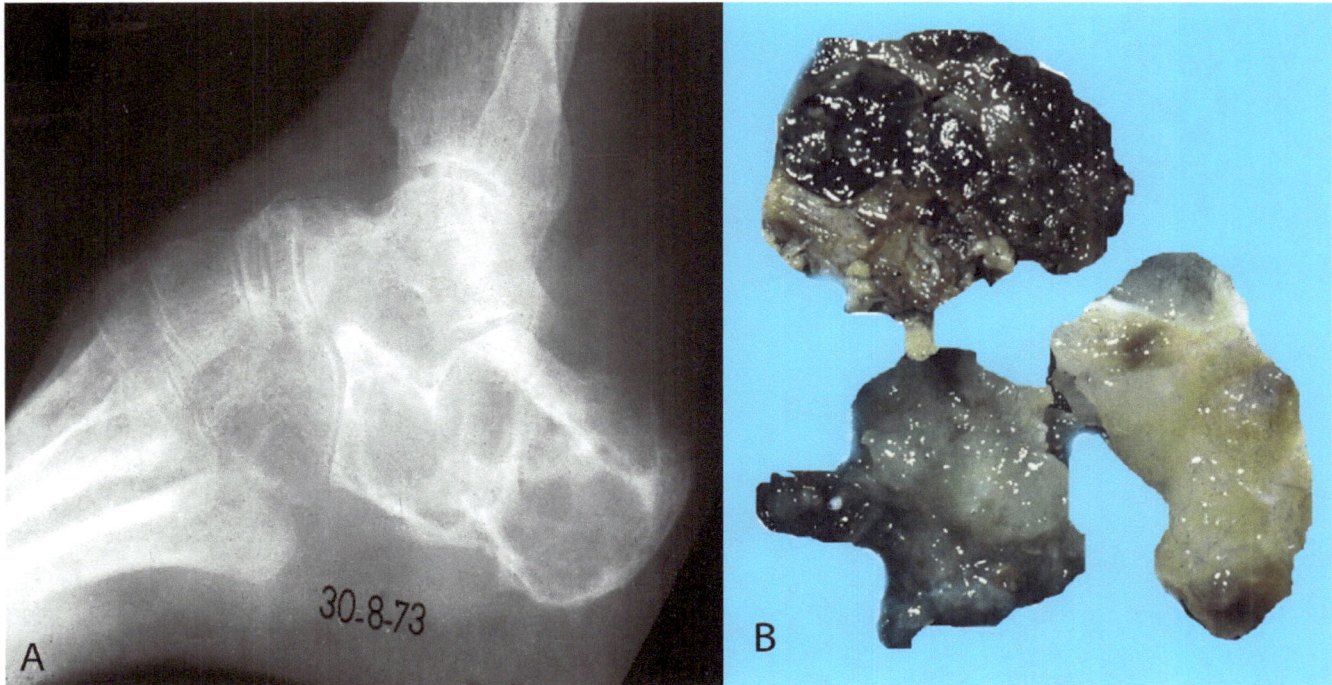

Fig. 2.17 Myxoid chondrosarcoma: (A) multicentric destructive lytic tumor in the calcaneum on x-ray; (B) gross appearance of a mucoid jelly like tumor mass.

Bumpass et al [40] reported a case of myxoid chondrosarcoma of phalanx, and found only 32 cases of skeletal myxoid chondrosarcoma in the literature. The case fulfilled criteria for intraosseous origin with proper radiographic findings. The most common sites for 32 cases were femur 28%, pelvis 19% and foot 16%. One case of skeletal myxoid chondrosarcoma presented in this paper showed the same chromosomal translocation as found in the extraskeletal tumor, and the authors believe that both skeletal and extraskeletal tumors should be considered as a single tumor type.

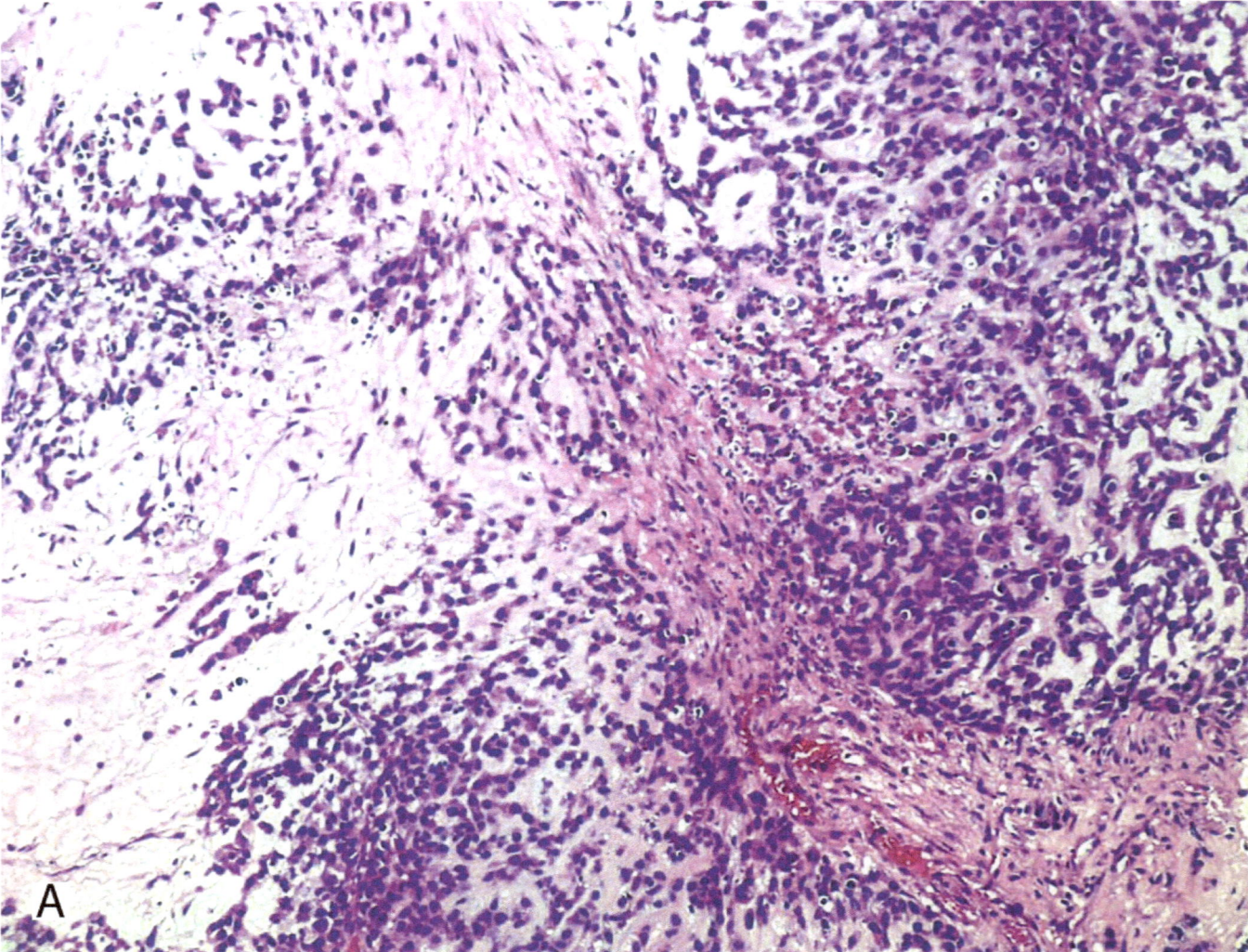

A

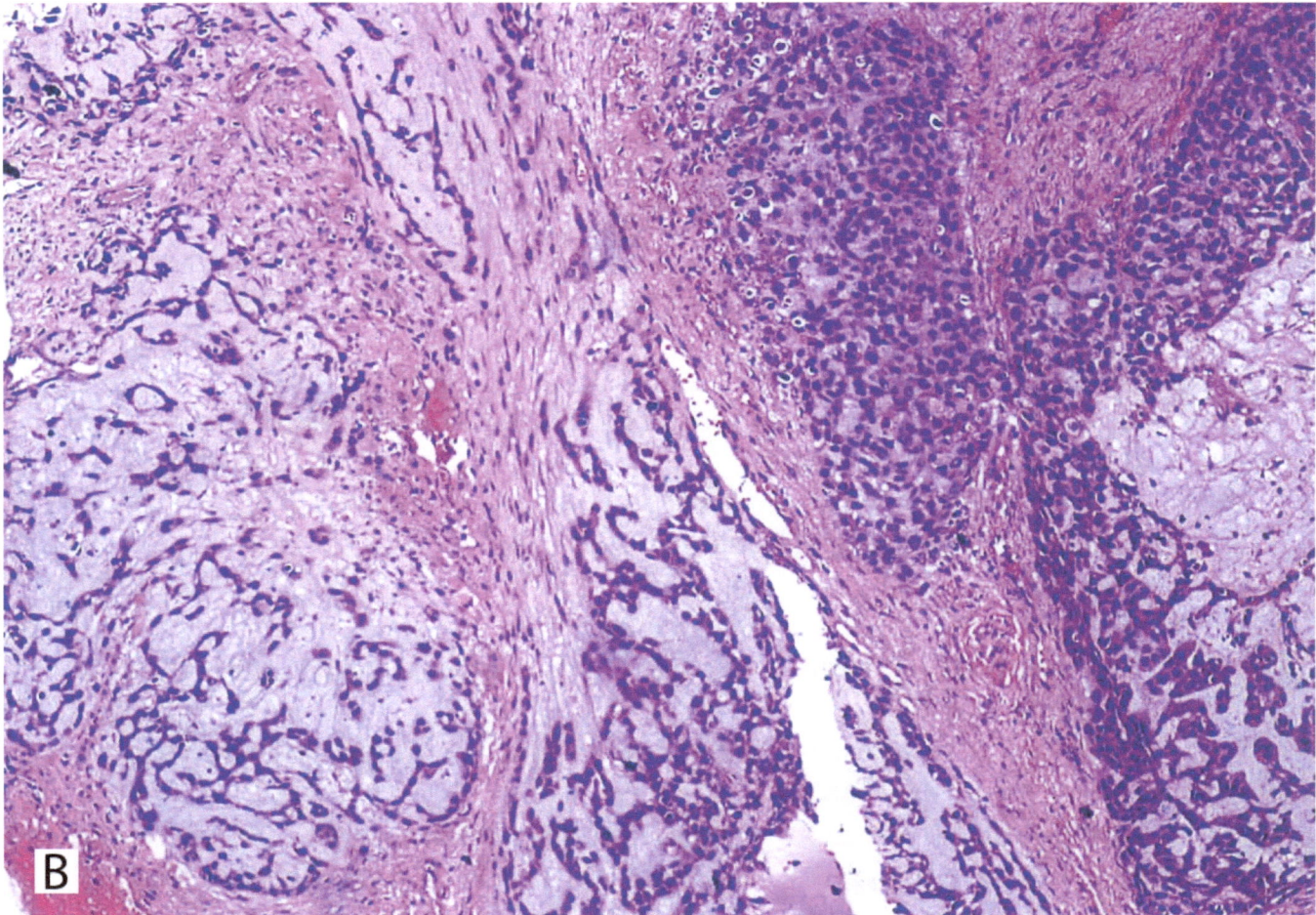

Fig. 2.18 Myxoid chondrosarcoma of bone: (A) Small cords, groups and sheets of small to medium sized neoplastic cells within a mild variable mucinous background; (B) cords of tumor cells widely separated by moderate amount of myxoid stroma.

References for Chapter 2

Osteochondroma

1. Schmale G.A., Coinrad E.U.III, Raskind W.H. (1994).The natural history of hereditary multiple exostoses.J.Bone.Joint Surg.Am.76:986-992.
2. Unni K K and Inwards C Y (2010) Osteochondroma. In: Dahlin's Bone tumors: general aspects and data on 10,165 cases. Sixth edition. Lippincott Williams & Wilkins, Philadelphia. pp 9-21
3. Ahmed, A.R. Tan, T.S., Unni, K.K., Collins, M.S., Wenger, D.E., and Sim, F.H. (2003). Secondary chondrosarcoma in osteochondroma: Report of 107 patients. Clin.Orthop. Relat. Res. 411:193-206.

Bizarre Parosteal Osteochondromatous Proliferation

4. Nora F E, Dahlin D C, Beabout J W 1983 Bizarre parosteal osteochondromatous proliferations of the hands and feet. Am J Surg Pathol 7: 245-250

5. Meneses MF, Unni KK, Swee RG: Bizarre parosteal osteochondromatous proliferation of bone (Nora's lesion). Am J Surg Pathol 1993; 17:691-7.

6. Gruber G, Giessauf C, Leithner A et al. Bizarre parosteal osteochondromatous proliferation (Nora lesion): a report of 3 cases and a review of the literature. Can J Surg. 2008 Dec; 51(6): 486–489.

Reactive periosteitis

7. Spjut HJ, Dorfman HD: Florid reactive periostitis of the tubular bones of the hands and feet: A benign lesion which may simulate osteosarcoma. Am J Surg Pathol 1981; 5:423-33.

Periosteal chondroma

8. Bauer T W, Dorfman H D, Latham J T Jr 1982 Periosteal chondroma: a clinicopathologic study of 23 cases. Am J Surg Pathol 6: 631-637

9. Nojima T, Unni K K, McLeod R A et al. 1985 Periosteal chondroma and periosteal chondrosarcoma. Am J Surg Pathol 9: 666-677

Chondroblastoma

10. Codman, E.A., "Epiphyseal chondromatous giant cell tumors of the humerus". Surg Gynecol Obstet, 52, 543-548, 1931.

11. Green P, Whittaker R P 1975 Benign chondroblastoma: case report with pulmonary metastasis. J Bone Joint Surg Am 57: 418-420

12. Kahn L P, Wood S M, Ackerman L V 1969 Malignant chondroblastoma: report of two cases and review of the literature. Arch Pathol Lab Med 88: 371-376

13. Jambhekar N A, Desai P B, Chitale D A et al. 1998 Benign metastasizing chondroblastoma: a case report. Cancer 82: 675-678

Chondromyxoid fibroma

14. Jaffe HL, Lichtenstein L. Chondromyxoid fibroma of bone: a distinctive benign tumor likely to be mistaken especially for chondrosarcoma. *Arch Path*. 1943. 19:541-51.

15. Wu C T, Inwards C Y, O'Laughlin S, Unni K K et al. 1998 Chondromyxoid fibroma of bone: a clinicopathologic review of 278 cases. Hum Pathol 29: 438-446

16. Baker A C, Rezeanu L, O'Loughlin S et al. 2007 Juxtacortical chondromyxoid fibroma of bone: a unique variant-a case study of 20 patients. Am J Surg Pathol 31: 1662-1668

17. Granter S R, Renshaw A A, Kozakewich H P et al. 1998 The pericentromeric inversion, inv (6)(p25q13), is a novel diagnostic marker in chondromyxoid fibroma. Mod Pathol 11: 1071-1074

Chondrosarcoma

18. Bovée J V, van der Heul R O, Taminiau A H et al. 1999 Chondrosarcoma of the phalanx: a locally aggressive lesion with minimal metastatic potential—a report on 35 cases and a review of the literature. Cancer 86: 1724-173

19.   Andreou D, Ruppin S, Fehlberg S et al. 2011 Survival and prognostic factors in chondrosarcoma: results in 115 patients with long-term follow-up. Acta Orthop 82: 749-755

20.   Björnsson J, McLeod R A, Unni K K et al. 1998 Primary chondrosarcoma of long bones and limb girdles. Cancer 83: 2105-2119

Secondary chondrosarcoma

21.   Ahmed A R, Tan T S, Unni K K et al. 2003 Secondary chondrosarcoma in osteochondroma: report of 107 patients. Clin Orthop Relat Res 411: 193-206

22.   Garrison R C, Unni K K, McLeod R A et al. 1982 Chondrosarcoma arising in osteochondroma. Cancer 49: 1890-1897

23.   Verdegaal S H, Bovée J V, Pansuriya T C et al. 2011 Incidence, predictive factors, and prognosis of chondrosarcoma in patients with Ollier disease and Maffucci syndrome: an international multicenter study of 161 patients. Oncologist 16: 1771-1779

24.   Liu J, Hudkins P G, Swee R G et al. 1987 Bone sarcomas associated with Ollier's disease. Cancer 59: 1376-1385

Dedifferentiated chondrosarcoma

25.   Dahlin D C, Beabout J W 1971 Dedifferentiation of low-grade chondrosarcomas. Cancer 28: 461-466

26.   Reith J D, Bauer T W, Fischler D F et al. 1996 Dedifferentiated chondrosarcoma with rhabdomyosarcomatous differentiation. Am J Surg Pathol 20: 293-298

27.   Littrell L A, Wenger D E, Wold L E et al. 2004 Radiographic, CT, and MR imaging features of dedifferentiated chondrosarcomas: a retrospective review of 174 de novo cases. Radiographics 24: 1397-1409

28.   Grimer R J, Gosheger G, Taminiau A et al. 2007 Dedifferentiated chondrosarcoma: prognostic factors and outcome from a European group. Eur J Cancer 43: 2060-2065

29.   Staals E L, Bacchini P, Bertoni F 2006 Dedifferentiated central chondrosarcoma. Cancer 106: 2682-2691

Clear cell chondrosarcoma

30.   Björnsson J, Unni K K, Dahlin D C et al. 1984 Clear cell chondrosarcoma of bone: observations in 47 cases. Am J Surg Pathol 8: 223-230

31.   Collins M S, Koyama T, Swee R G et al. 2003 Clear cell chondrosarcoma: radiographic, computed tomographic, and magnetic resonance findings in 34 patients with pathologic correlation. Skeletal Radiol 32: 687-694

32.   Unni KK, Dahlin DC, Beabout JW, Sim FH: Chondrosarcoma: clear-cell variant. A report of sixteen cases. J Bone Joint Surg Am 1976; 58:676-83.

33.   Itälä A, Leerapun T, Inwards C et al. 2005 An institutional review of clear cell chondrosarcoma. Clin Orthop Relat Res 440: 209-212

Mesenchymal chondrosarcoma

34. Nakashima Y, Unni K K, Shives T C et al. 1986 Mesenchymal chondrosarcoma of bone and soft tissue: a review of 111 cases. Cancer 57: 2444-2453

35. Shakked R J, Geller D S, Gorlick R et al. 2012 Mesenchymal chondrosarcoma: clinicopathologic study of 20 cases. Arch Pathol Lab Med 136: 61-75

36. Lee A F, Hayes M M, Lebrun D et al. 2011 FLI-1 distinguishes Ewing sarcoma from small cell osteosarcoma and mesenchymal chondrosarcoma. Appl Immunohistochem Mol Morphol 19: 233-238

37. Harwood AR, Krajbich JI, Fornasier VL: Mesenchymal chondrosarcoma: a report of 17 cases. Clin Orthop Relat Res 1981; 158:144-8.

Myxoid chondrosarcoma

38. Enzinger FM, Shiraki M Extraskeletal myxoid chondrosarcoma. An analysis of 34 cases. Hum Pathol 1972; 3:421-435

39. Antonescu CR, Argani P, Erlandson RA, et al Skeletal and extraskeletal myxoid chondrosarcoma: a comparative clinicopathologic, ultrastructural, and molecular study Cancer 1998; 83:1504-1521

40. Bumpass, DB, Kyriakos M, Rubin DA, Manske, et al, "Myxoid chondrosarcoma of the phalanx with an EWS translocation: A case report and review of the literature. J Bone and Joint Surg 2011; 93,6. e23 1-7

Chapter 3: Osseous (bone forming) tumors

Osteoblastoma (and osteoid osteoma)

The tumor currently known as 'osteoblastoma' was first described by Lichtenstein in 1952 as 'osteogenic fibroma of bone'. Later in 1954 Dahlin and Johnson [1] reported 11 cases of this tumor under the name 'giant osteoid osteoma' to emphasize its similarity to osteoid osteoma. The currently accepted name 'osteoblastoma' was used first by both Lichtenstein [2] and Jaffe [3] separately in 1956 'as a category of osteoid-and bone-forming tumors other than classical osteoid osteoma.

Definition

Osteoblastoma, as understood now, is a locally aggressive intramedullary bone forming tumor with histology similar to that of benign osteoid osteoma. Despite the histological similarity, osteoid osteoma and osteoblastoma are two distinct tumors clinically, radiologically and prognostically. Osteoid osteoma is a limited growth potential nidus, which is about less than 1.5 cm. in diameter; while osteoblastoma is locally aggressive, and may grow up to 15 cm in diameter [4]

Clinical findings

While osteoid osteomas occur in children and adolescents, majority of osteoblastoma occur in the age groups 10 to 30 years.

The vertebral column including sacrum is the most frequent site. The other sites involved include long bones, mainly upper and lower end of femur, and upper end of tibia. Mandible and tarsal bones are other bones involved. Osteoid osteoma presents with pain which is typically relieved by non-steroidal anti-inflammatory agents. Pain in osteoblastoma is milder, and ceases to respond to anti-inflammatory agents after prolonged therapy. Neurological symptoms may be associated with tumors occurring in the spine. Rarely the tumor may be associated with systemic symptoms of fever, anorexia and weight loss, and may show generalized periosteitis. The systemic symptoms disappear on excision of the tumor.

X--ray

Osteoid osteoma shows the nidus surrounded by a sclerotic zone; this sclerotic zone is absent in osteoblastoma. Osteoblastoma presents as a well-defined lytic lesion with or without sclerotic border. The radiologic features may be nonspecific, and not uncommonly overlap with those of osteosarcoma (Fig. 3.1 A, B, C, D).

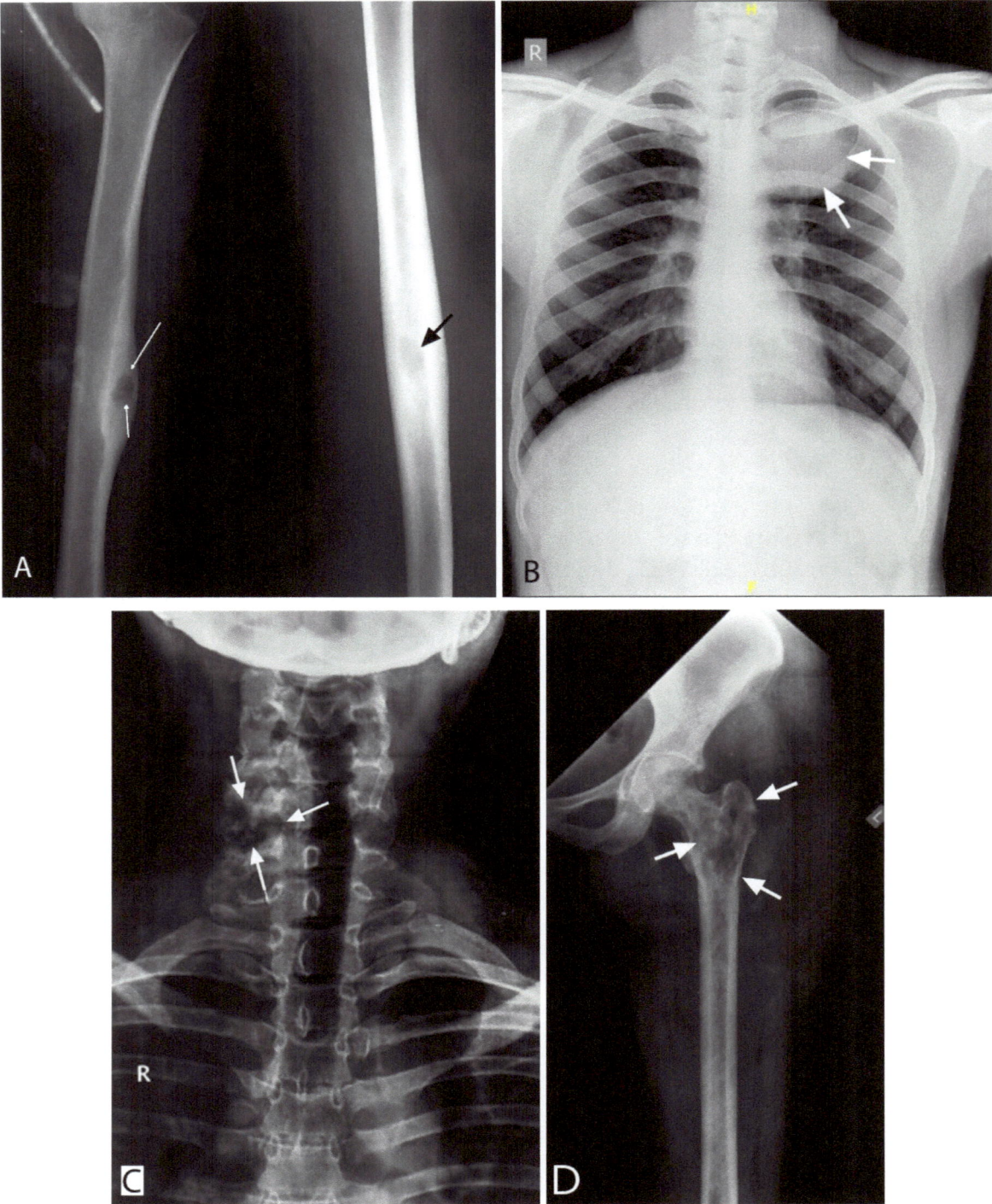

Fig. 3.1 Osteoid osteoma and osteoblastoma: (A) typical radiological features of osteoid osteoma for comparison; (B) Large slightly opaque round lesion destroying proximal second rib (arrows); (C) small destructive lesion of cervical vertebra (arrows); (D) a partly well-defined osteolytic lesion (arrows)of trochanter, proved to be Osteoblastoma on histology.

Gross

The tumor is soft to gritty and greyish pink; appears well circumscribed in resected specimens and may have a shell of reactive bone.

Microscopic

Osteoblastoma shows anastomosing trabeculae of woven bone or osteoid rimmed by one to two layers of 'osteoblasts' with loosely arranged fibrovascular stroma filling the intertrabecular spaces. The lesional bone producing cells are quite plump with dark staining large nuclei. There is usually no nuclear atypia, nor atypical mitoses. The lesional cells have been called 'osteoblasts' only to distinguish them from osteocytes of Haversian canals. At places osteoblasts may form contiguous sheets. (Fig.3.2 A, B, C). The trabeculae may show varying degree of mineralization. Rarely cartilage may be seen in osteoblastoma. Not uncommonly there may be associated aneurysmal bone cyst –like change resulting in massive expansion of the tumor. [5,6,7,8] Mirra et al. have reported a case of pseudomalignant osteoblastoma with bizarre pleomorphic nuclei which despite the alarming nuclear features had a benign course. [9]

Prognosis

Though majority of osteoblastomas behave in benign fashion and some regress spontaneously, few behave in aggressive manner (aggressive osteoblastoma). The latter are characterized by epithelioid osteoblasts with sheet-like growth pattern. It is not possible to predict behavior of the tumor. In fact, the aggressive nature is more often recognized by behavior than by morphology. For this reason it is now advised that all osteoblastomas be called as such without the prefix 'benign'[5,10]

With limited biopsy material it may not be possible to distinguish osteoblastoma from osteosarcoma. Areas of necrosis, sheets of epithelioid osteoblasts and mitoses particularly atypical ones indicate malignancy. It may be noted that osteoblastoma and osteosarcoma are not related entities and osteoblastoma does not transform to osteosarcoma.

Filippi et al [11] reported 26 cases of 'epithelioid multinodular osteoblastoma' a variant characterized by male predominance. Jaw was the most commonly affected site. Histologically it was characterized by multinodular growth pattern with epithelioid osteoblasts, often in sheets. Some of these tumors showed histological features of aggressive behavior, but till now all have had benign course.

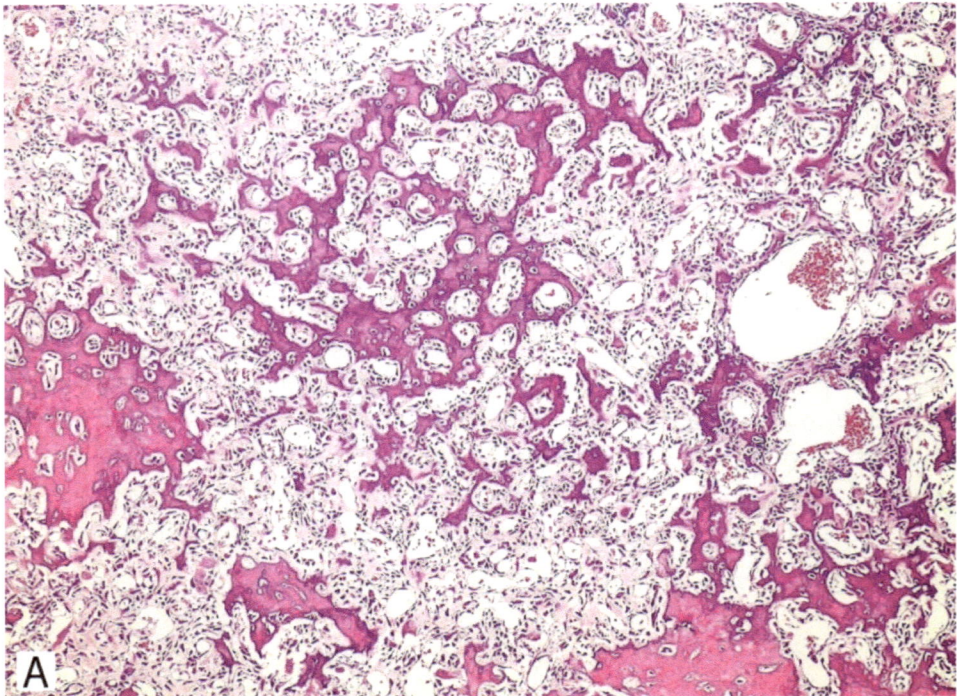

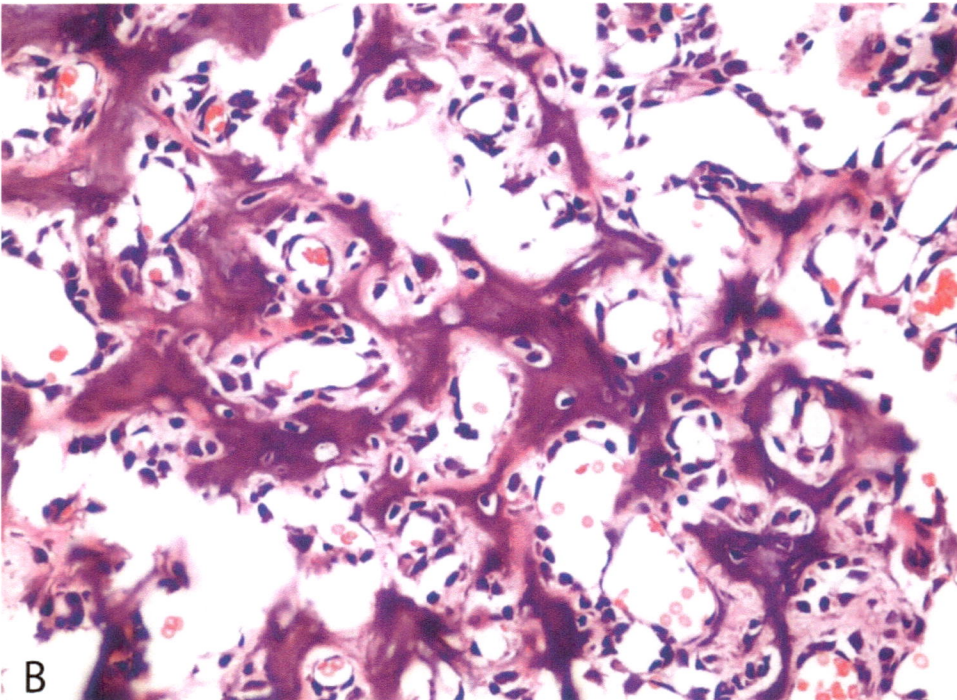

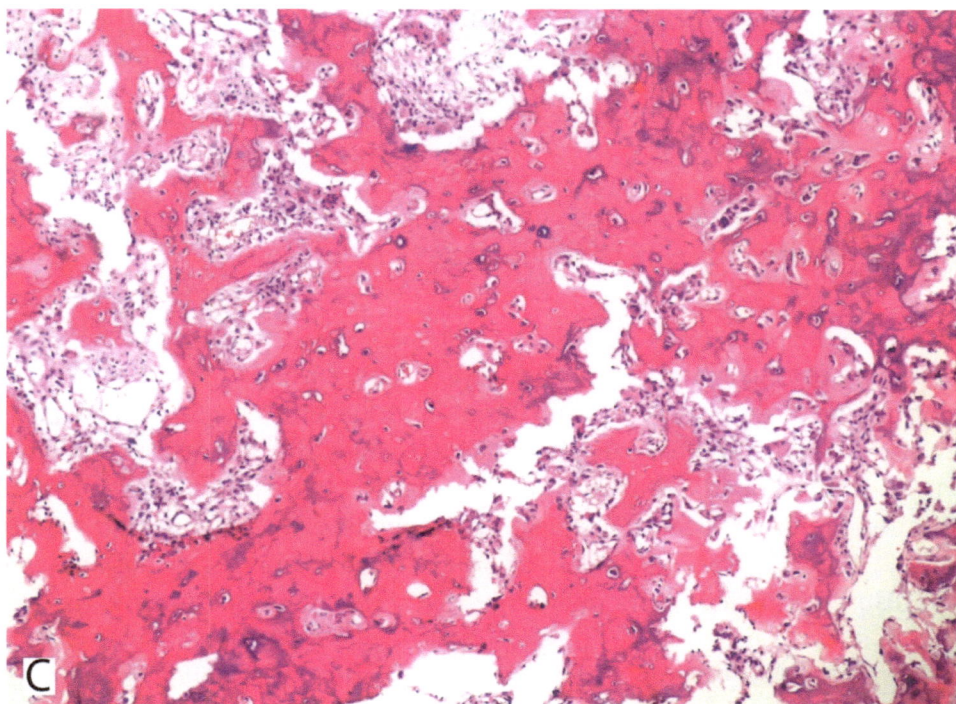

Fig. 3.2 (A) low power view of osteoblastoma showing anastomosing thick trabeculae of woven bone separated by vascular spindle cell stroma, Note one or two layers of prominent osteoblasts in the trabeculae; (B) high power of picture in A, note lack of any nuclear atypia or mitotic activity; (C) there is overabundant development of well-formed osteoid of type and extent, which is never seen in conventional osteosarcoma

Osteosarcoma

Conventional osteosarcoma is a high grade primary intramedullary sarcoma of bone with potential to form osteoid.

Clinical findings

While osteosarcoma may arise in any bone, majority occur in the metaphysis of long tubular bones. The common sites are lower end of femur, upper end of tibia and upper end of humerus. These sites represent most actively growing bone ends and together account for 60% of the cases. About 90% of osteosarcomas occur in the metaphysis, while only 9 % occur in diaphysis. [12] Rarely epiphysis may be involved. The tumor shows bimodal age distribution: majority occur in adolescents and young adults, the peak incidence being in the second decade. The remaining occurs in persons above age 40 years. [13] Osteosarcoma in children younger than five years is rare.

Primary osteosarcomas occur in bones with no underlying predisposing pathology. Most of the conventional high grade osteosarcomas that occur in the adolescents and young adults are primary tumors; while those that occur secondary to some predisposing pathology, like radiation therapy or Paget's disease of bone, are seen in older individuals.

The incidence of secondary osteosarcoma in Paget disease is estimated to be 1%. Paget disease associated osteosarcoma accounts for more than 50% cases in patients aged more than 60 years.[12] Almost 70% of the secondary osteosarcomas in western countries are associated with Paget's disease.

Post-radiation osteosarcoma now occurs rarely because of improved radiation techniques. [14,15] Other rare predisposing causes include bone infarcts, metallic implants, osteochondroma, fibrous dysplasia, and chronic osteomyelitis.[13]

Clinical features

Pain and swelling are the commonest symptoms. Not uncommonly some injury may draw attention to the swelling. Rarely tumor presents with pathologic fracture.

Radiological findings

Plain X-ray picture of osteosarcoma is varied, depending on extent of the disease, bone destruction and mineralization of the tumor osteoid. The tumor may be either osteoblastic, osteolytic, or as is more often the case, mixed osteoblastic and osteolytic. Usually the tumor is seen filling the medullary cavity, infiltrating the cortex and reaching the periosteum. Periosteum offers resistance to tumor infiltration. As the periosteum is lifted up, there is reactive new bone deposition resulting in 'Codman triangle' (Fig.3.3 A, B, C, D, E). This is evidence of bone destruction and extraosseous extension of the tumor. The tumor also extends along the medullary cavity replacing the marrow tissue. This extension may not be contiguous.

While X-rays are best suited to diagnose the destructive nature and evidence of bone production by the tumor, MRI is ideal to determine the extent of disease pre-operatively. This information is of great importance to the surgeon in planning treatment.

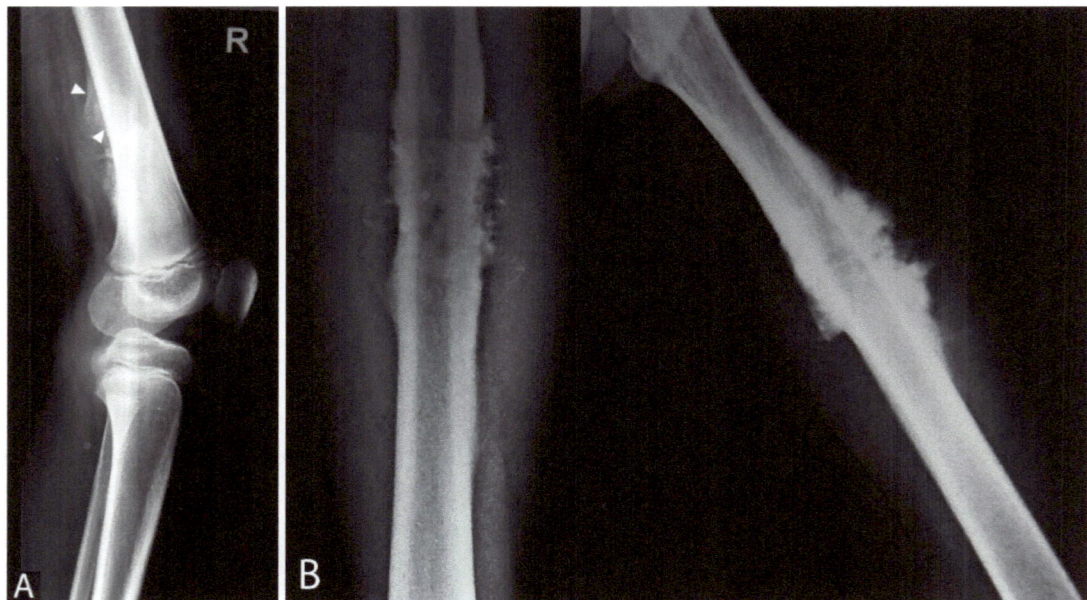

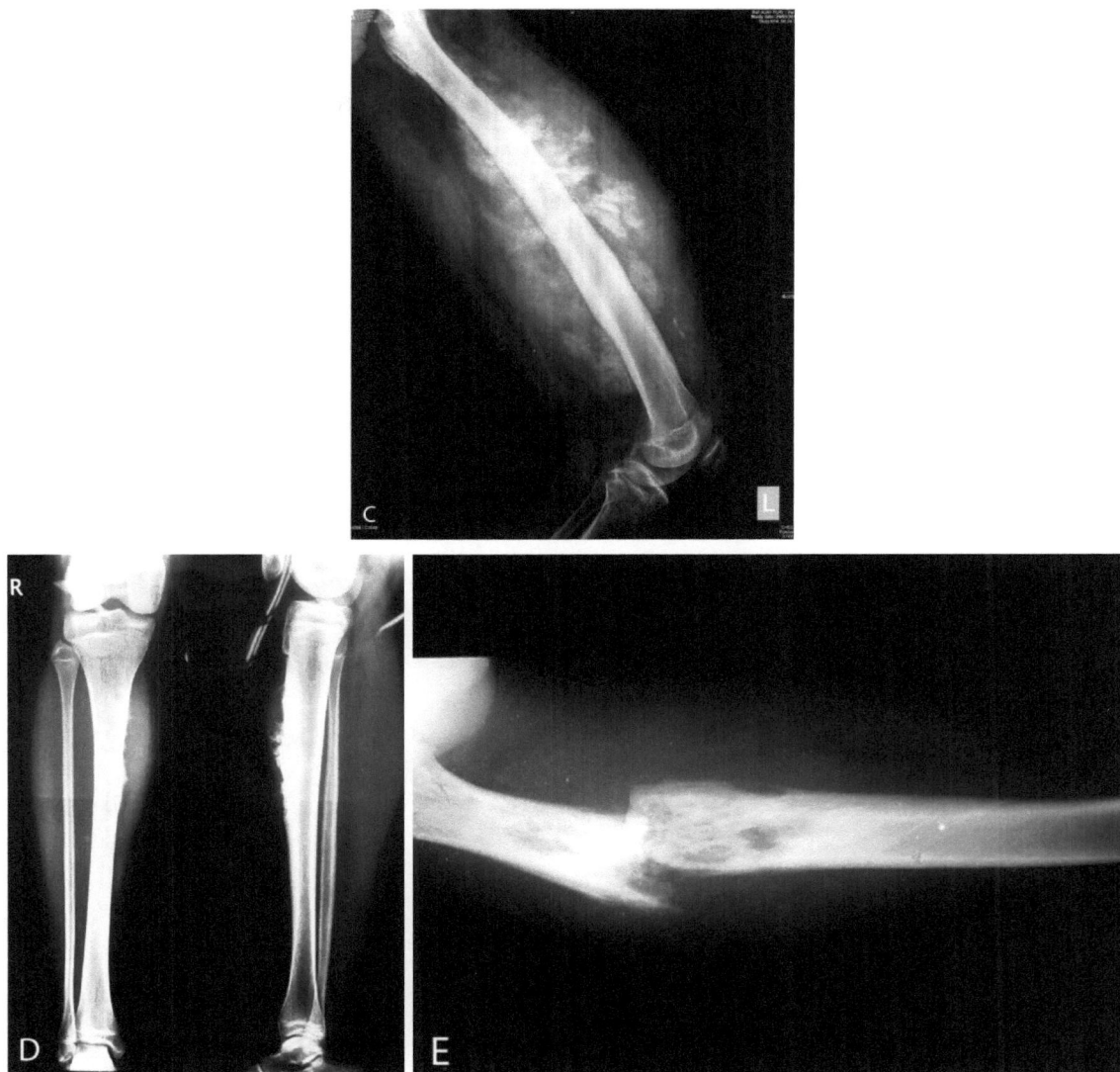

Fig. 3.3 Osteosarcoma: (A) intramedullary osteosarcoma showing Codman's triangle (arrow heads) (B) surface osteosarcoma with high grade morphology, cortex not destroyed ; (C) Osteosarcoma involving diaphysis of femur with a soft tissue component; (D) Osteosarcoma upper end of tibia with lifting of periosteum and soft tissue component; (E) Osteosarcoma upper end of femur with pathological fracture.

Gross appearance of the tumor shows destruction of the host bone and expansion of bone contours. The consistency depends on amount of bone, cartilage and fibrous tissue. The tumor is fleshy, greyish white and firm. The tumor with significant chondroblastic component appears greyish, glistening. There may be necrosis and hemorrhage. Tumor extends in to the soft tissues forming eccentric or circumferential mass.

Histological picture of conventional osteosarcoma is dominated by high grade sarcoma and tumor osteoid. In addition, there may be malignant chondroid and fibroblastic components. The tumor cells are described as spindle shaped, oval, round, plasmacytoid, epithelioid and rarely clear cell. [13, 16, 17]

Demonstration of osteoid, in however small quantity, establishes histogenetic diagnosis of osteosarcoma. Osteoid that is in direct contact with malignant cells is apparently formed by the tumor cells, and hence called 'tumor osteoid'. On H&E stained sections unmineralized osteoid appears as dense eosinophilic amorphous hyaline extracellular material that is not unlike collagen. Not uncommonly, it is difficult to distinguish unmineralized osteoid from extracellular collagen. Non-osteoid collagen appears fibrillary, the fibrils arranged in linear, parallel rows. Mineralization is evidence that the structure most probably is osteoid.

Depending on the presence of the predominant type of matrix, the cases may be classified as osteoblastic, chondroblastic or fibroblastic osteosarcomas. None of these types have prognostic relevance.

Osteoblastic / sclerosing

Majority of osteosarcomas are osteoblastic, and osteoid may be deposited in thin intercellular, lace-like or filigree pattern. In sclerosing variant there is abundant osteoid with sparse neoplastic cells which may at times be inconspicuous (Fig.3.4 A, B, C, D, E, F). It needs to be emphasized that diagnosis of malignancy in sclerosing osteosarcoma is made on the basis of cytology of neoplastic cells, while the subtyping is based on the amount and type of osteoid.

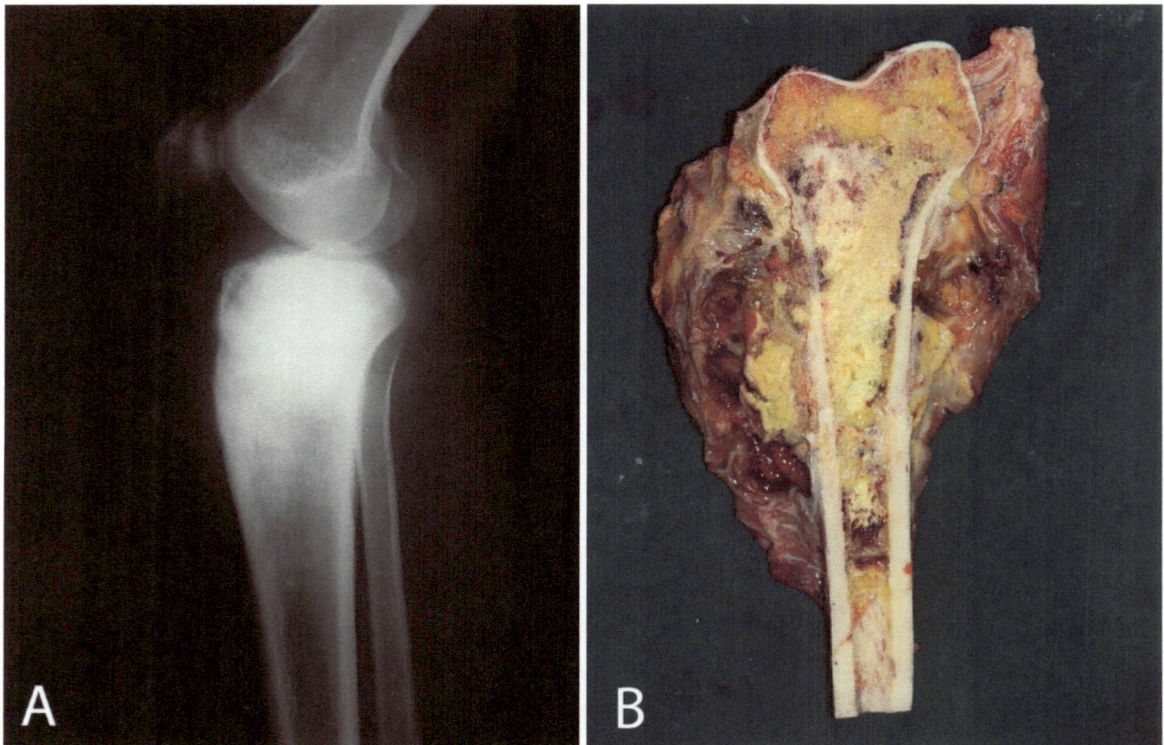

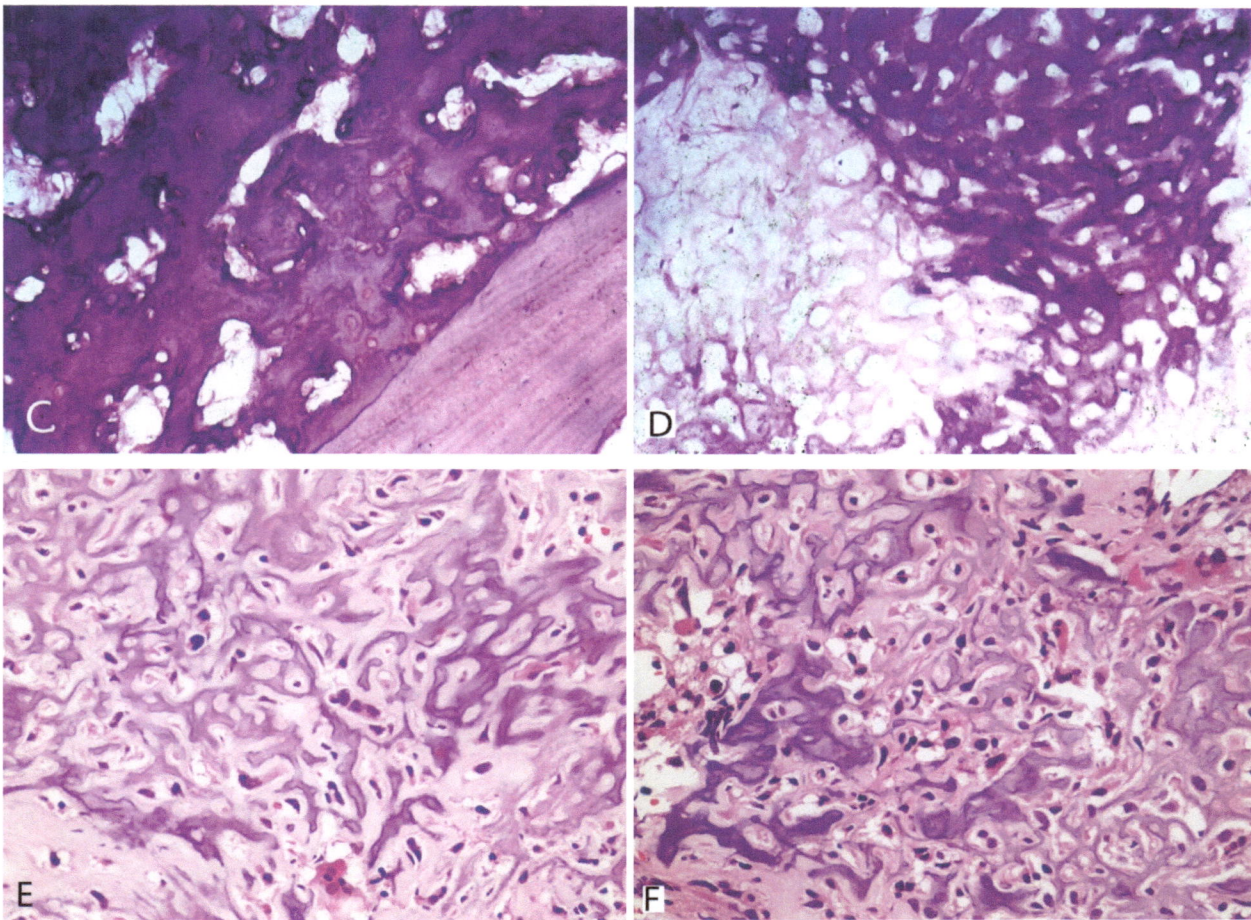

Fig. 3.4 Sclerosing osteosarcoma: (A) diffuse opacity at upper end of tibia; (B) a solid yellowish white growth in upper end of tibia, tumor extends beyond the cortex into the soft tissues; (C) dense heavily mineralized basophilic thick trabeculae containing few scattered hardly visible neoplastic cells, note host bone, lower right; (D) large areas of acellular hyalinized matrix; E&F) abundant basophilic sclerotic bone with fewer neoplastic cells in (E); more neoplastic cells within sclerotic tumor bone in (F).

There are different patterns of osteoid deposition which pathologists should be aware of. These patterns have no prognostic significance. It is mineralized osteoid which imparts radiological densities. A predominantly osteoblastic tumor with unmineralized osteoid appears radiolucent, making its recognition as osseous tumor difficult.

Chondroblastic Osteosarcoma

Chondroblastic component in these tumors is highly malignant (Fig. 3.5 A, B, C, D) and demonstration of osteoid in the tumor matrix may be difficult, especially in limited biopsy material. Patient's young age, site of involvement and radiological features should alert the pathologist to the possible diagnosis of osteosarcoma; [18] This has great therapeutic relevance.

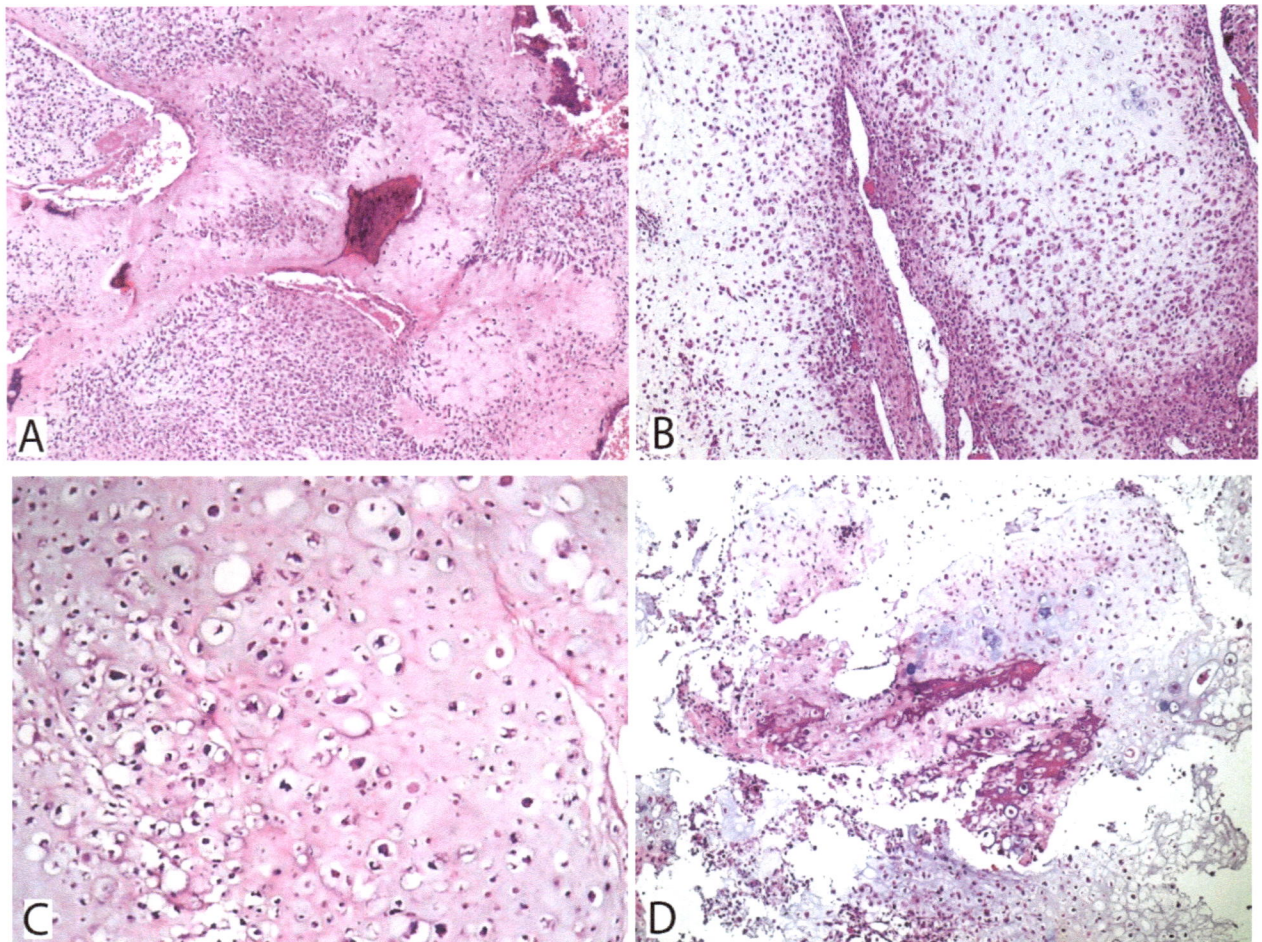

Fig. 3.5 (A, B, C, D) variable appearance of chondroblastic osteosarcoma, the lesion can be mistaken for a proper conventional chondrosarcoma of adults.

Fibroblastic osteosarcoma

About 25% of the osteosarcomas are predominantly fibroblastic and spindle cellular with close resemblance to high grade fibrosarcoma (See figure 5.3 in Chapter 5) with variable stromal collagen. Osteoid is usually sparse in these cases. Less commonly the pattern may be reminiscent of Undifferentiated high grade pleomorphic sarcoma (Malignant fibrous histiocytoma). In such cases even when osteoid is difficult to demonstrate, diagnosis of osteosarcoma is justified in proper clinical setting and radiological context.

Giant cell rich osteosarcoma

Scattered benign looking multinucleated osteoclast-like giant cells are not uncommon in conventional osteosarcomas. Rarely these cells may predominate the histological picture making distinction between giant cell tumor and osteosarcoma difficult or even impossible (Fig. 3.6 A, B, C). Young age of the patient, metaphyseal location of the tumor and radiological features point towards the correct diagnosis. Careful search for nuclear atypia and osteoid matrix should be undertaken. [17]

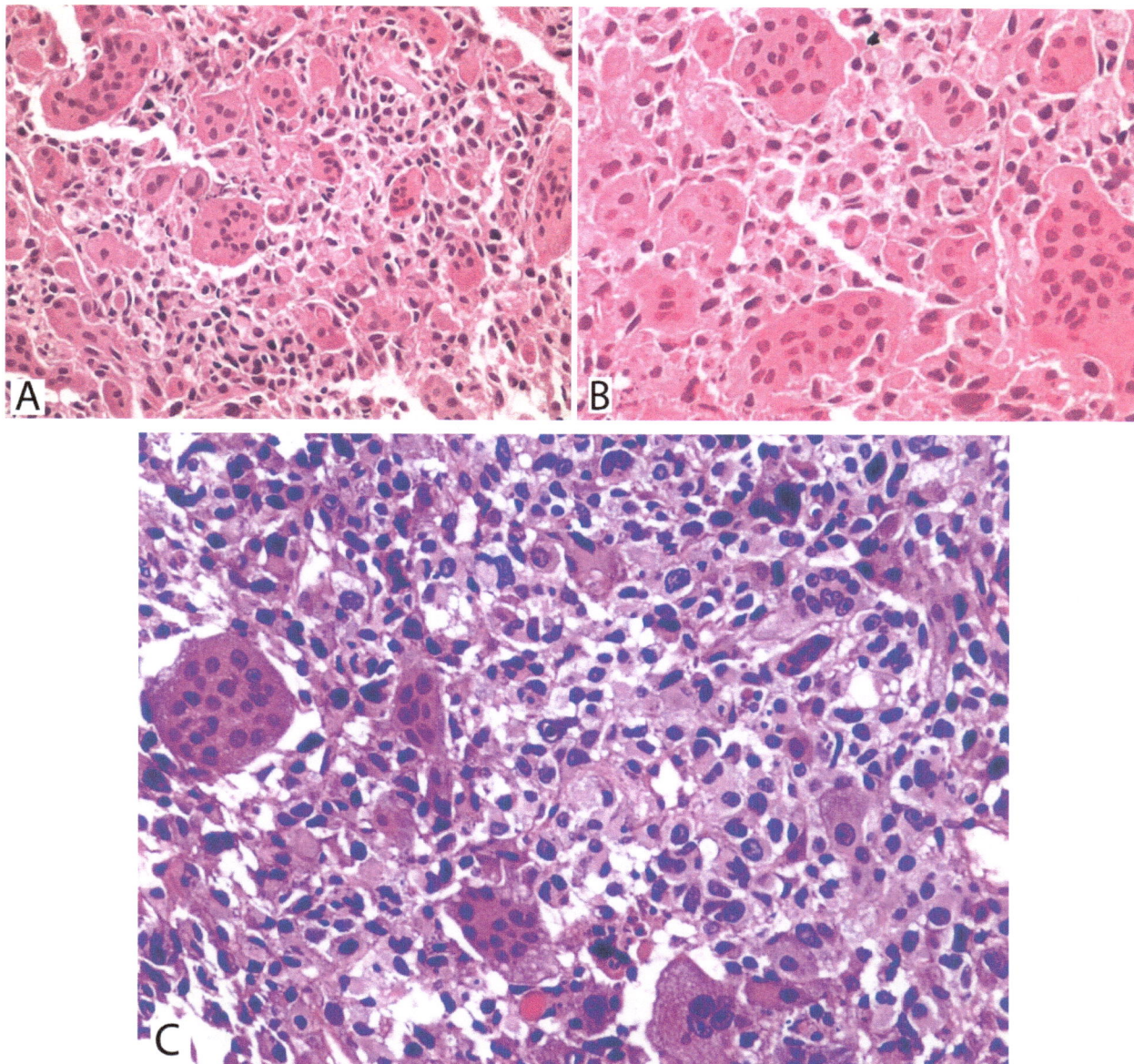

Fig. 3.6 Giant cell rich osteosarcoma: (A, B, C) all pictures share a large number of osteoclasts but the intervening cells display prominent nuclear anaplasia, particularly marked in picture (C)

Epithelioid type osteosarcoma

Rarely conventional osteosarcoma may show epithelial phenotype *(Fig.3.7)* raising possibility of metastatic carcinoma. If diagnosis of metastatic carcinoma on histology is entertained in a young patient and given that x-ray picture is appropriate, possibility of osteosarcoma should be seriously considered. [19]

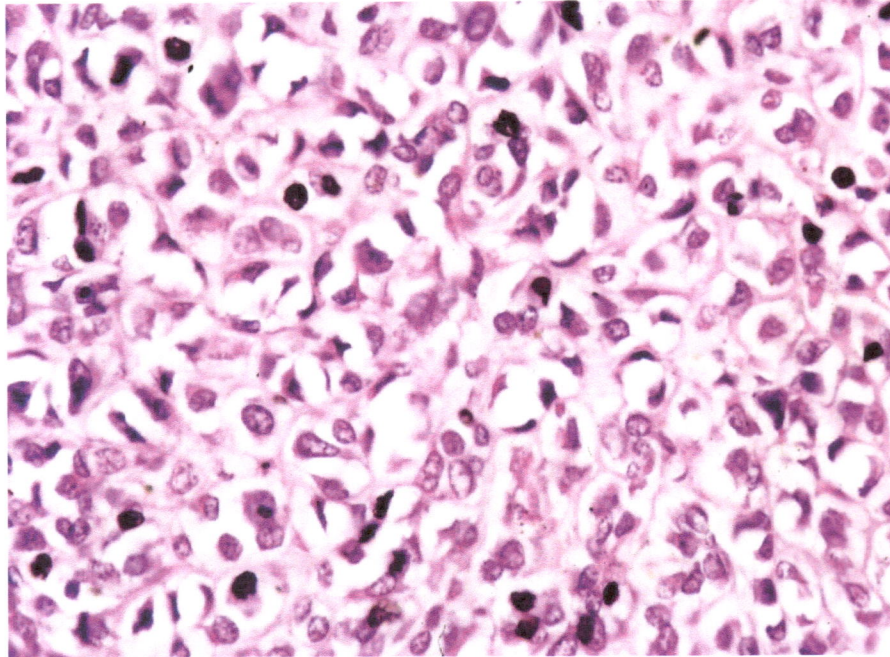

Fig. 3.7 "Epithelioid" osteosarcoma: large vacuolated epithelioid cells in contiguous sheets; this was a 28-year old patient with a large tumor mass in the metaphysio diaphyseal region of femur, clinical presentation suggested diagnosis of osteosarcoma. Immunohistochemically the tumor cells were negative for epithelial markers ruling out metastatic carcinoma.

Conventional osteosarcoma is high grade malignant tumor, and if untreated grows aggressively at the local site with frequent and early hematogenous spread and fatal outcome. Metastasis occurs most often to lungs and bones (Fig. 3.7).

The modern limb saving surgery techniques and pre- operative chemotherapy regimen have greatly improved prognosis of osteosarcoma. With effective chemotherapy five-year disease free survival has been reported to be as high as 80%. [20, 21, 22, 23, 24]

Telangiectatic osteosarcoma

Is telangiectatic osteosarcoma malignant counterpart of aneurysmal bone cyst, or is it a cystic change occurring in conventional high grade osteosarcoma? It is now accepted as distinct clinico-pathologic entity because of its radiological and histological features.[25, 26] The lesion is often misinterpreted as aneurysmal bone cyst, grossly and radiologically. Some presenting features and age incidence are not different from those of conventional osteosarcomas.

X-ray

Radiologically, the tumor appears as radiolucent, aneurysmal bone cyst-like lesions. Some of them may even show fluid levels on MRI imaging. Presence of sclerosis negates diagnosis of telangiectatic osteosarcoma. [27]

Gross

Telangiectatic osteosarcoma presents as predominantly expansile cystic lesion. The tumor appears cystic, hemorrhagic and spongy mass with little solid component.
Characteristically, it is described as 'bag of blood' (Fig. 3.8 A, B).

Microscopic

This is a blood filled multiloculated cystic lesion and the septa separating the cystic areas may show atypical cells with or without osteoid material. These atypical cells may at times be sparse and may be missed altogether. There may be just blood clots with a few isolated malignant spindle cells floating within. Awareness that high grade osteosarcoma may present predominantly as multicystic mass should alert the Pathologist to look for atypical cells. This tumor is highly sensitive to modern chemotherapy but prognosis remains the same as for any conventional osteosarcoma (Fig. 3.8 C, D). [28]

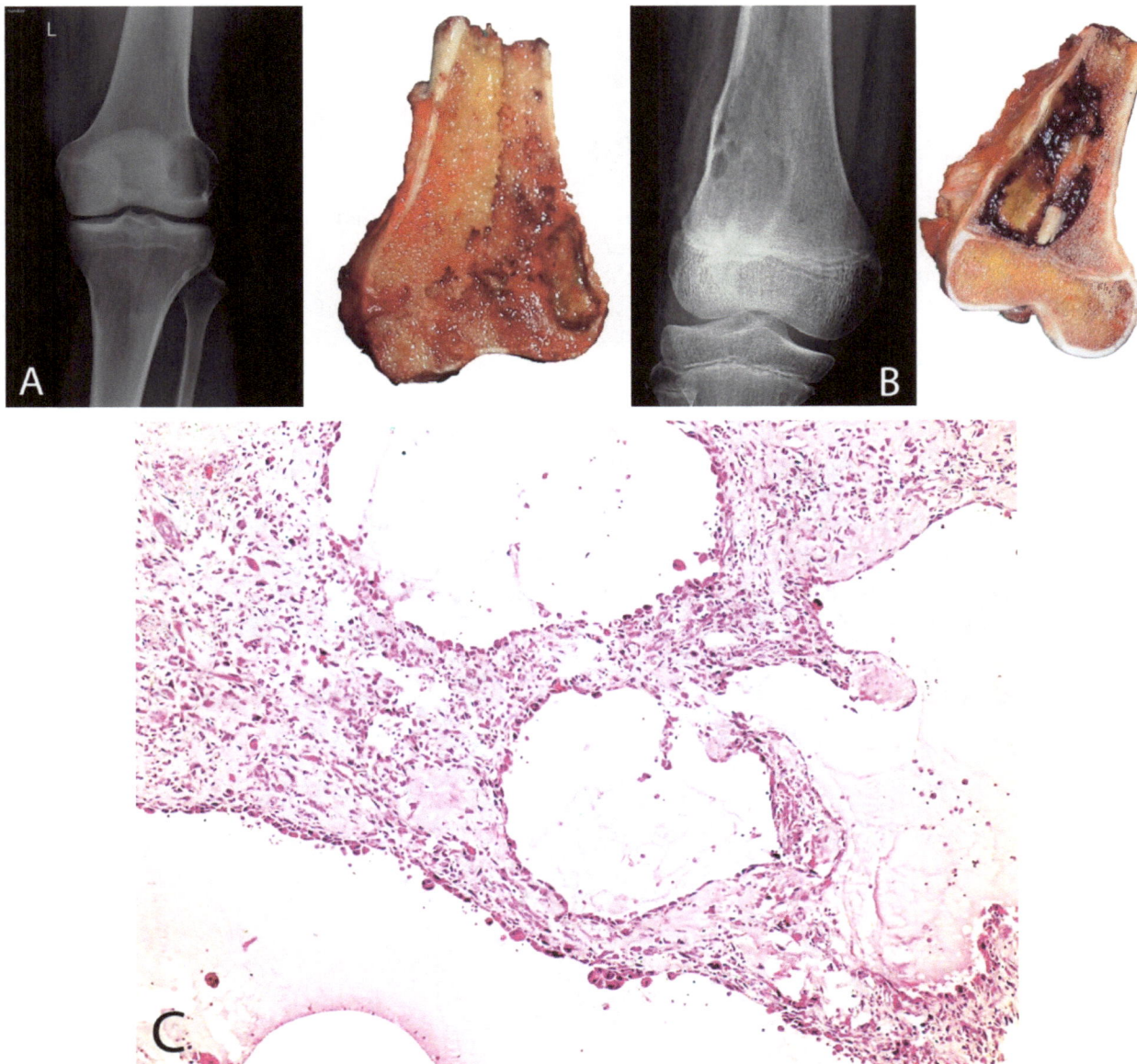

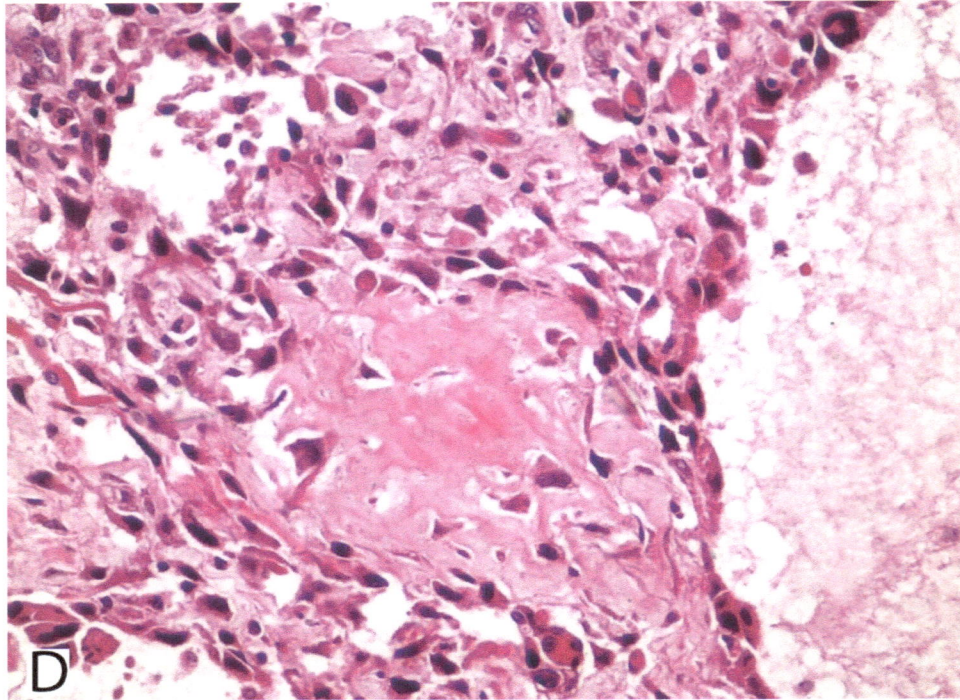

Fig. 3.8 Telangiectatic osteosarcoma (A) X- ray of lower part of left femur shows a well circumscribed lytic lesion in the epiphysis ; resected tumor bearing femur reveals a cystic lesion filled with hemorrhagic tumor; (B) a similar X ray showing circumscribed lytic lesion in the metaphysis and distal diaphysis containing small cysts ; gross specimen shows cystic tumor filled with blood clots, note fragments of grafted bone in the earlier conservative surgery; (C) large cysts separated by neoplastic osteoblasts in sheets, and osteoid; (D) high magnification to show malignant osteoblasts and tumor osteoid in the cyst wall.

Small cell osteosarcoma

This variant of osteosarcoma may be mistaken for other small round cell tumors like Ewing sarcoma and lymphoma. Clinical and radiological features of small cell osteosarcoma are similar to those of conventional osteosarcoma. The tumor is composed of small round cells, like those in Ewing sarcoma and malignant lymphoma (Fig. 3.9 A, B, C, D). Detection of tumor osteoid should lead to correct diagnosis, although this is not possible in all cases.

The prognosis of this tumor is no different from that of conventional osteosarcomas. [29, 30, 31]

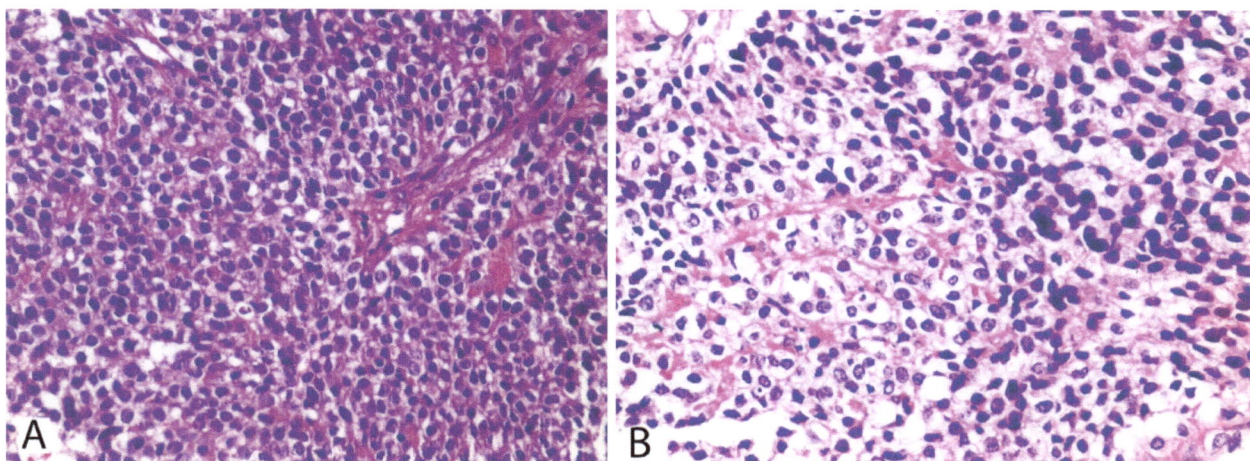

Fig. 3.9 Small cell osteosarcoma (A) sheets of small round malignant cells; (B) streaks of osteoid matrix forming a cobweb;

Prognosis of osteosarcoma

There have been great advances in treatment of osteosarcoma. Pre-operative chemotherapy with limb salvage surgical procedures have greatly improved long term survival to almost 80% compared to prognosis of 20% in pre-chemotherapy era.[22, 23] Response to pre-operative chemotherapy remains the most reliable prognostic indicator of long term survival. For this reasons it is advocated that resected specimens be thoroughly examined in systematic manner for percentage of "tumor necrosis".[24, 32] More than 90% "tumor necrosis" is thought to be indicator of good prognosis, while less than 90 % tumor necrosis is thought to be poor indicator of survival.[22]

Post-chemotherapy tumor necrosis assessment

Extent of tumor regression following chemotherapy is the most important prognostic factor. Pathologists are called upon to assess the extent of tumor 'necroses in resected specimens of osteosarcoma following neoadjuvant chemotherapy. The specimen should be stripped off the total soft tissue component. A thin slice of the whole specimen can be cut out with an electrical saw. The area of the grossly identifiable tumor may be marked out, and cut in several smaller pieces, and processed. Estimate of percentage of total tumor necroses and viable tumor can be calculated.[32]

'Necrosis' of more than 90% of the tumor following chemotherapy is thought to be an indicator of good prognosis. With appropriate change in chemotherapy, significant number of non-responders may be salvaged.[22]

Low grade intraosseous (central) osteosarcoma

Intraosseous low grade osteosarcoma is intraosseous counterpart of parosteal osteosarcoma. In 1977 Unni et al [33] from Mayo clinic reported a series of 27 cases and drew attention to this entity. Essentially this is an intraosseous low grade spindle cell tumor which produces abundant new bone in the form of parallel rows of branching and interconnecting trabeculae of well-formed lamellar bone, features similar to those of parosteal osteosarcoma. The tumor cells are bland with minimal or mild nuclear atypia. Mitosis is rare or absent. Occasional islands of cartilage and mature fat may be seen within the tumor. Also seen are scattered multinucleated giant cells.[34]

Clinical findings

These are often mistaken for benign conditions, if proper attention is not paid to subtle radiological features suggesting aggressive behavior. The tumor forms about 1 % of all osteosarcomas, peak age incidence being in second and third decades. Males and females are affected equally. The tumors present with pain and swelling. Some tumors may remain asymptomatic for years. Lower end of femur, upper end of tibia and upper end of humerus are common sites. It typically involves metaphysis. Flat bones like pelvis, scapula and skull are involved infrequently.[13]

X-ray

Plain X rays show heavily mineralized and well marginated tumor Fig.3.10 A, B) Features of aggressiveness may be subtle or altogether absent.

Microscopic

Not uncommonly, low grade osteosarcoma is mistaken for fibrous dysplasia. The cells in fibrous dysplasia are short, spindle or stellate shaped with uniformly distributed stromal collagen in the background. Bone is characteristically short curvilinear, or psammomatous. On the other hand, in low grade osteosarcoma the cells are longer and more compactly arranged with mild nuclear atypia and occasional mitosis; and bone trabeculae are lamellar and arranged in branching, intercommunicating parallel rows.

These are low grade (grade 1), slowly growing; and wide local excision proves curative in most cases. Incomplete removal may result in recurrence; recurrent tumor may show higher grade (grade 2). [13, 34]

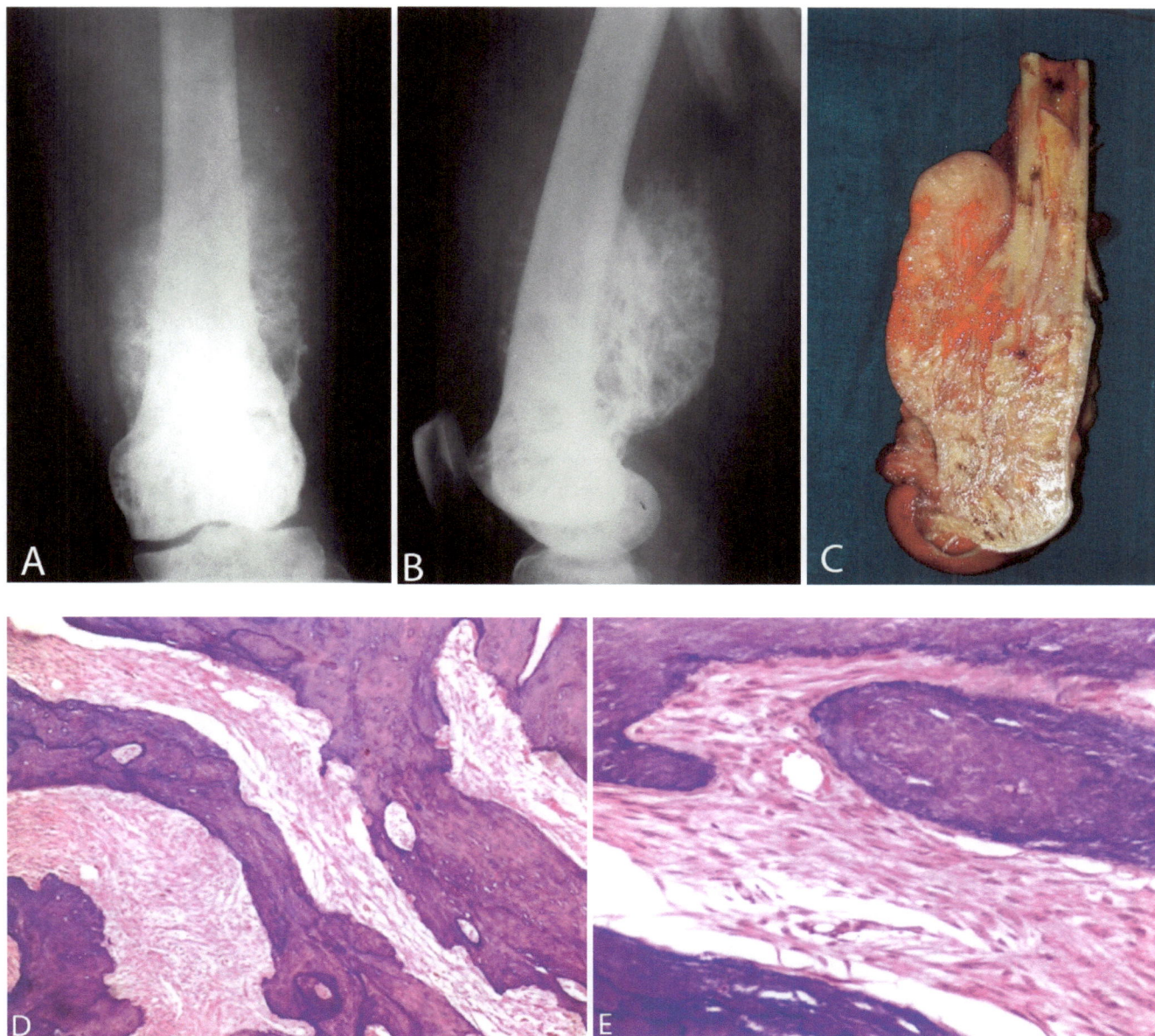

Fig 3.10; (A and B) X ray of the lower femur showing permeative pattern involving the distal diaphysis and epimetaphyseal region with an intraosseous and extra-osseous osteoid tumor; (C) Gross specimen of intraosseous tumor extending in to the soft tissue; (D, E) neoplastic woven/ lamellar bone trabeculae with mildly cellular spindle cells fascicles with intervening collagen, nuclear atypia is minimal.

Parosteal osteosarcoma

Clinical findings

Both intraosseous low grade osteosarcoma and parosteal osteosarcoma are same tumors; one occurs in the medullary cavity, and the other, on the surface of bone. Parosteal osteosarcoma forms 4% of all osteosarcomas in Mayo Clinic series.[35] There is slight female predominance and majority occurs in second and third decades.

The tumor typically occurs on the surface of the long tubular bone, growing along posterior aspect of the lower end of femur (Fig 3.11 A, B) and upper end of tibia. Upper end of humerus, pelvis, scapula and skull bones are involved rarely.

Pain, swelling and restriction of movements are the common presenting symptoms.

X-ray

The features are characteristic: heavily mineralized tumor with broad base on the surface and occurrence at the metaphyseal or meta-diaphyseal locations. CT/ MRI may show cortical involvement. The tumor may surround the bone. There may be complete or incomplete lucent zone between the tumor and the cortex.

Gross

The tumor is greyish white, fibrous, firm to gritty. Soft, fleshy areas, when present, represent dedifferentiated component.

Microscopic

Histology is similar to that of intraosseous well differentiated osteosarcoma. It is hypocellular, composed of spindle fibrous cells arranged in compact fascicles, and parallel rows of branching and interconnecting mature lamellar bone trabeculae. These bone trabeculae may be surrounded by osteoblasts. Not uncommonly islands of hyaline cartilage may be seen on the outer surface of the tumor as a cartilaginous cap mimicking osteochondroma, or within the main tumor. There is only nuclear atypia, and rare mitosis. The tumor invades the marrow cavity, or the soft tissue. (Fig.3.11C, D) ; and Fig.3.12 B-C) [36]

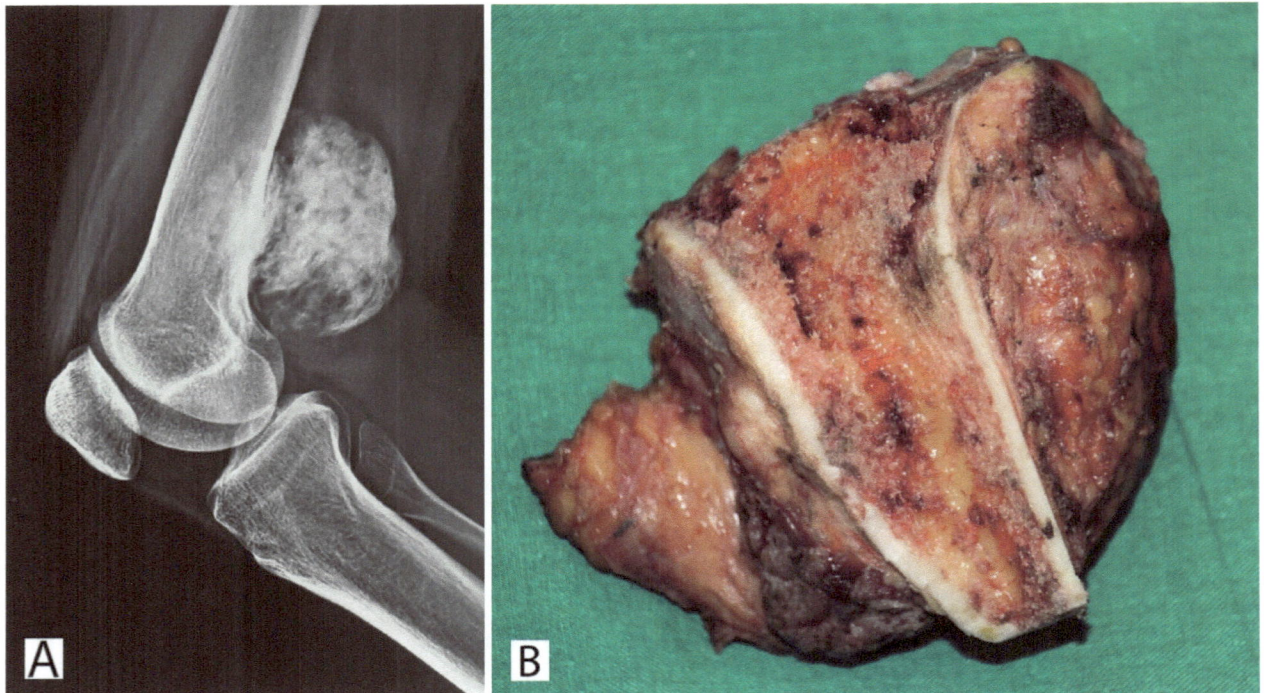

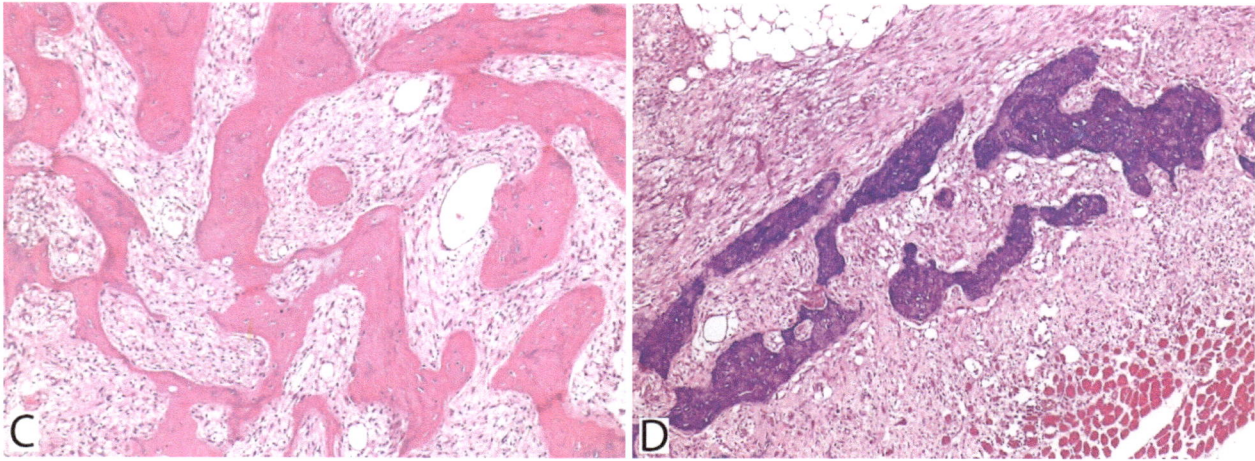

Fig. 3.11 Parosteal osteosarcoma (A) lateral view of lower femur with a large osteoid tumor on the surface , extending in to the surrounding soft tissue : (B) limb-saving surgery: resected lower femur, note intact uninvolved cortex; (C) irregularly thick osteoid trabeculae with cement lines, and intervening moderately cellular spindle cell population; (D) invasion of calcified neoplastic trabeculae and spindle cell component infiltration in the fat and muscle.

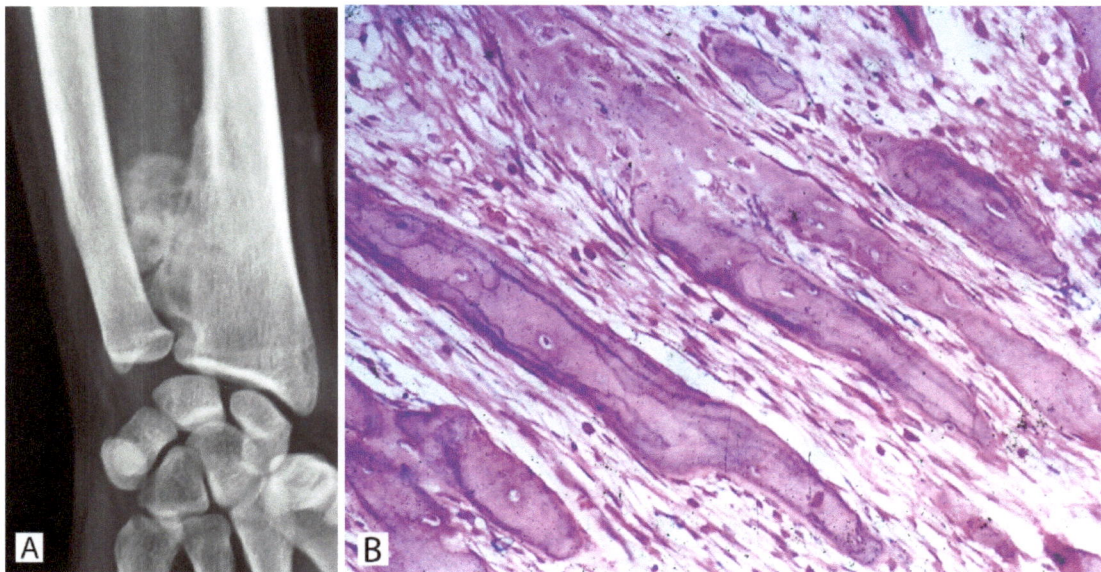

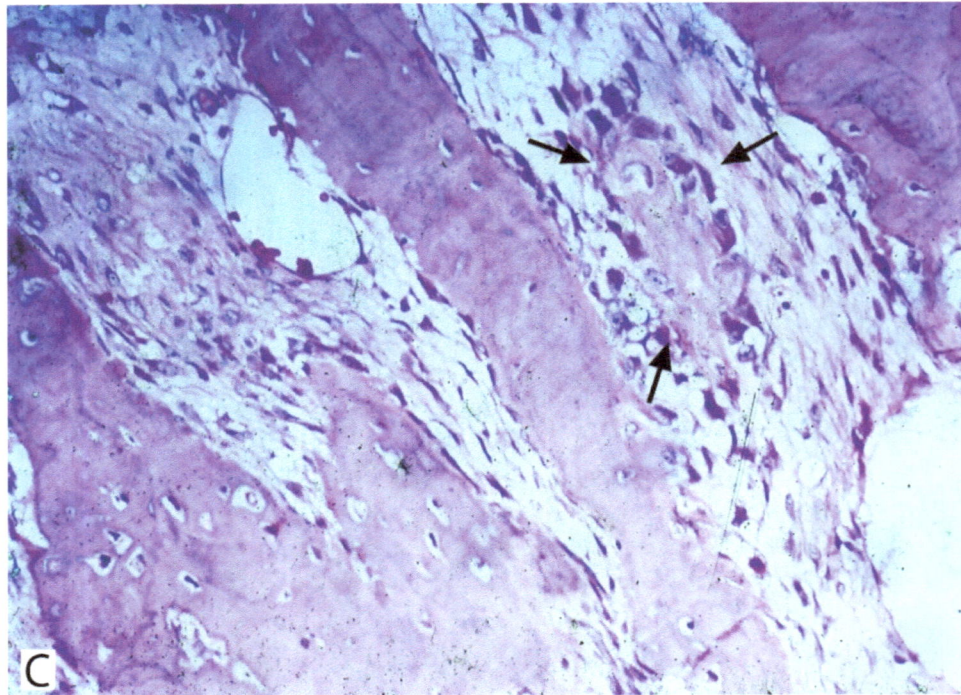

Fig. 3.12 (A) osseous tumor on the surface of distal end of radius and mimicking osteochondroma, note cortical erosion and thickened periosteum; (B) parallel arrays of irregular woven bone trabeculae with cement lines, (C) same field but with a single trabeculum lined by very plump atypical osteoblasts (arrows).

The tumor is usually graded as grade 1 on scale of 1 to 4. In about 20%, the tumor is more cellular and nuclei more atypical qualifying for grade 2 lesions. The recurrent tumor may show higher grade. About 15% of the tumors show dedifferentiation in to high grade sarcoma, usually osteosarcoma, fibrosarcoma or Undifferentiated high grade pleomorphic sarcoma (Malignant fibrous histiocytoma) .[37, 38]

Total extirpation is the treatment of choice, which usually results in five-year survival of more than 90%.[35, 36] Dedifferentiated tumors behave more aggressively, like grade 4 tumors, resulting in metastasis and death.[37, 38]

Periosteal osteosarcoma

Clinical findings

Periosteal osteosarcoma is a rare intermediate grade tumor that occurs on surface of bone and displays predominant chondroblastic morphology. Peak incidence is in the second and third decades, with slight male predominance. The tumor occurs on long tubular bone, most common bones involved being femur, tibia and humerus. Clavicle, ribs, mandible, pelvis and skull are involved rarely.[13] Pain, swelling and restriction of movements are the common symptoms.

Radiology

X ray shows irregularly mineralized tumor on the surface. Calcified spicules are seen within the tumor perpendicular to the cortical surface. The underlying cortex may be thickened and breached. The tumor infiltrates into the soft tissues. CT and MRI are essential to assess the extent of tumor invasion. The tumor often encircles the long tubular bones.

Gross

Grossly, it is a large, fusiform mass involving part or entire circumference of the bone shaft. The tumor has significant cartilaginous component in the form spicules that run perpendicular to the cortex. Cartilage component is ossified heavily near the cortex, being less ossified at the periphery.

Microscopic

Histologically periosteal osteosarcoma is intermediate grade chondroblastic osteosarcoma (Fig. 3.13 A, B). The cartilaginous part at the base shows endochondral ossification, which may then appear like mature bone. At the periphery, the tumor is spindle cellular with brisk mitotic activity. Lace like stromal osteoid may be seen at the periphery as evidence that this is indeed an osteosarcoma. [39]

Prognosis

The prognosis of this tumor is good with overall 5- and 10- year survival being 89% and 83% respectively. [40, 41, 42]

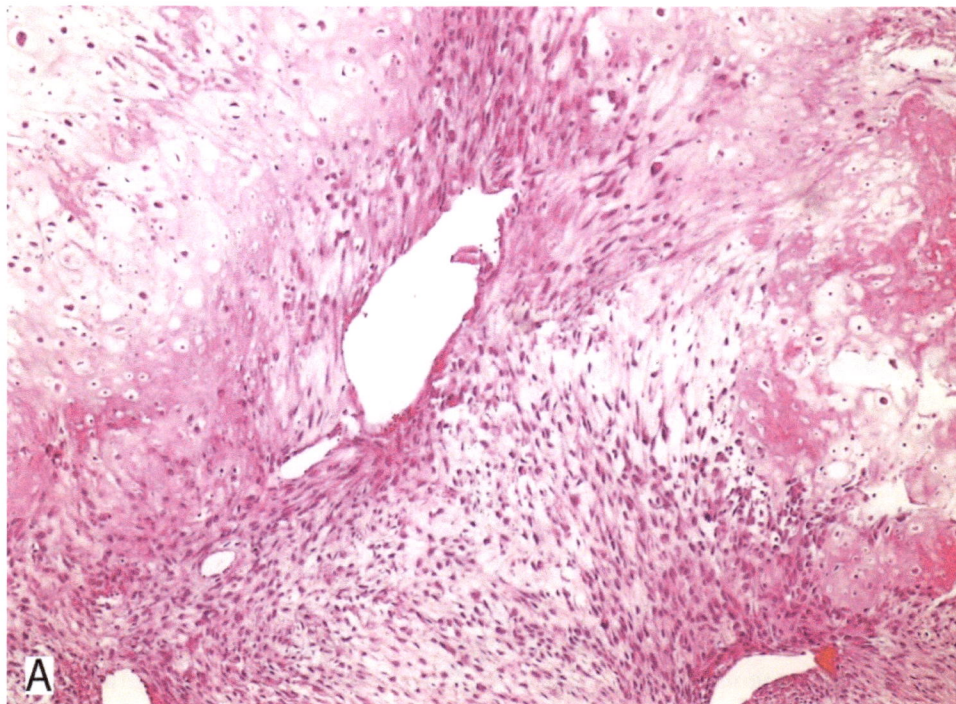

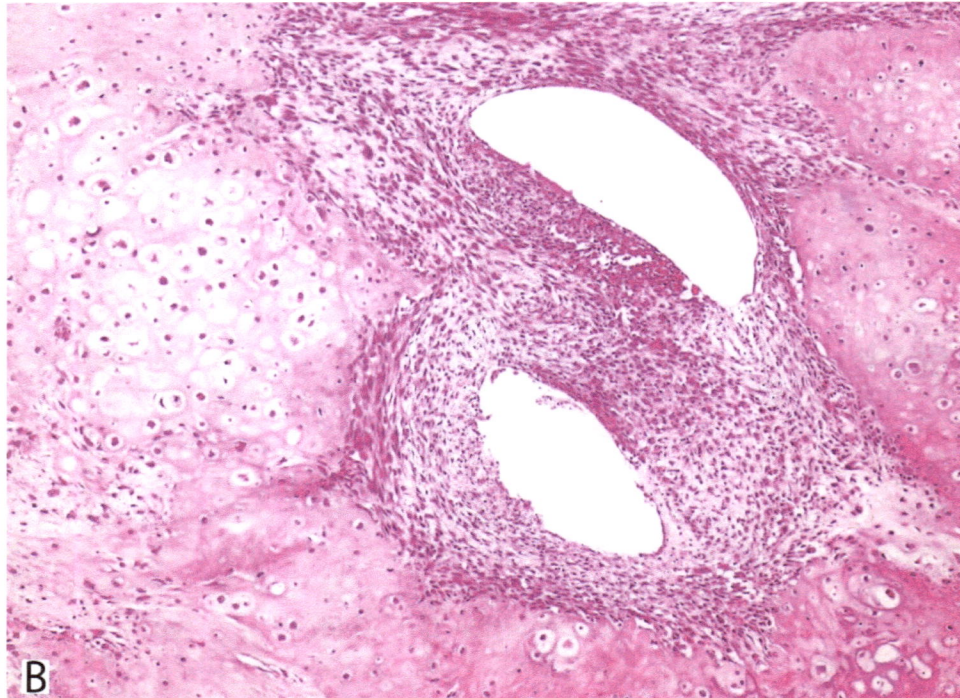

Fig. 3.13 (A, B) Periosteal osteosarcoma showing central cellular spindle cell component and hypocellular chondroid islands at the periphery

Prognosis

The prognosis of this tumor falls between parosteal osteosarcoma and high grade surface osteosarcoma (conventional osteosarcoma). The tumor has potential to recur when not excised totally, and even metastasize. Recurrence rate is said to be 70%.

High grade surface osteosarcoma

This is high grade osteosarcoma that occurs on the surface of bone with clinical and morphological features similar to those of conventional high grade tumors. The X-ray shows the tumor on the surface with cortical destruction and invasion in to the medullary cavity. Treatment options and prognosis are also the same as those of conventional osteosarcoma.[43, 44, 45]

References for Chapter 3

Osteoblastoma

1. Dahlin D C, Johnson E W Jr. Giant osteoid osteoma. J Bone Joint Surg Am. 1954; 36:559-572
2. Lichtenstein L Benign osteoblastoma; a category of osteoid-and bone-forming tumors other than classical osteoid osteoma, which may be mistaken for giant-cell tumor or osteogenic sarcoma. Cancer. 1956 Sep-Oct;9(5):1044-52.
3. Jaffe H L. Benign osteoblastoma. Bull Hosp Jt Dis. 1956; 17:141-151

4. Dorfman H D, Weiss S W. Borderline osteoblastic tumors: problems in the differential diagnosis of aggressive osteoblastoma and low-grade osteosarcoma. Semin Diagn Pathol. 1984; 1:215-234.
5. Marsh BW, Bonfiglio M, Brady LP et al. Benign osteoblastoma: range of manifestations. J Bone Joint Surg Am. 1975; 57:1-9.
6. Bertoni F, Donati D, Bacchini P et al. The morphologic spectrum of osteoblastoma (OBL): is its aggressive nature predictable? (abstract). Lab Invest. 1992; 66:3A.
7. Lucas D R, Unni K K, McLeod R A et al. Osteoblastoma: clinicopathologic study of 306 cases. Hum Pathol. 1994; 25:117-134
8. Della Rocca C, Huvos A G. Osteoblastoma: varied histological presentations with a benign clinical course: an analysis of 55 cases. Am J Surg Pathol. 1996; 20:841-850.
9. Mirra J M, Kendrick R A, Kendrick R E. Pseudomalignant osteoblastoma versus arrested osteosarcoma: a case report. Cancer. 1976; 37:2005-2014
10. Unni K K, Inwards C Y. Osteoblastoma. In: Dahlin's bone tumors: general aspects and data on 10,165 cases. Philadelphia, Lippincott Williams Wilkins, 2009;98-121.
11. Filippi R Z, Swee R G, Kr, Unni K K. Epithelioid multinodular osteoblastoma: a clinicopathologic analysis of 26 cases. Am J Surg Pathol. 2007; 31:1265-1268

Conventional osteosarcoma

12. Rosenberg A E, Cleton-Jansen A-M, Pinieux G de et al. Conventional osteosarcoma in WHO Classification of tumors of soft tissue and bone, Fourth edition. World Health Organization, Geneva. 2013; pp.282-288.
13. Unni K K, Inwards C Y. Osteosarcoma. In: Dahlin's Bone tumors: general aspects and data on 10,165 cases. Sixth edition. Lippincott Williams & Wilkins, Philadelphia. 1994:122-157.
14. Shaheen M, Deheshi B M, Riad S et al. Prognosis of radiation-induced bone sarcoma is similar to primary osteosarcoma. Clin Orthop Relat Res. 2006; 450:76-81.
15. Weatherby R P, Dahlin D C, Ivins J C. Postradiation sarcoma of bone: review of 78 Mayo Clinic cases. Mayo Clin Proc. 198; 56:294-306.
16. Dahlin D C, Coventry M B. Osteogenic sarcoma: a study of six hundred cases. J Bone Joint Surg Am. 1967; 49:101-110
17. Dahlin D C, Unni K K. Osteosarcoma of bone and its important recognizable varieties. Am J Surg Pathol. 1977; 1:61-72

Chondroblastic osteosarcoma

18. Bacchini P, Inwards C, Biscaglia R et al. Chondroblastoma like osteosarcoma. Orthopedics. 1999.22:337-339

Epithelioid osteosarcom

19. Deyrup A T, Montag A G. Epithelioid and epithelial neoplasms of bone. Arch Pathol Lab Med 2007; 131:205-216.

High-grade osteosarcoma

20. Bielack S S, Kempf-Bielack B, Delling G etal. Prognostic factors in high-grade osteosarcoma of the extremities or trunk: an analysis of 1,702 patients treated on neoadjuvant cooperative osteosarcoma study group protocols. J Clin Oncol. 2002; 20:776-790.

21. Hauben E I, Weeden S, Pringle J et al. Does the histological subtype of high-grade central osteosarcoma influence the response to treatment with chemotherapy and does it affect overall survival? A study on 570 patients of two consecutive trials of the European Osteosarcoma Intergroup. Eur J Cancer. 2002; 38:1218-1225

22. Ferrari S, Smeland S, Mercuri M et al Neoadjuvant chemotherapy with high-dose ifosfamide, high-dose methotrexate, cisplatin, and doxorubicin for patients with localized osteosarcoma of the extremity: a joint study by the Italian and Scandinavian Sarcoma G roups. J Clin Oncol. 2005; 23:8845-8852.

23. Bacci G, Longhi A, Versari M et al. Prognostic factors for osteosarcoma of the extremity treated with neoadjuvant chemotherapy: 15-year experience in 789 patients treated at a single institution. Cancer. 2006; 106:1154-1161

24. Whelan J S, Jinks R C, McTiernan A et al Survival from high-grade localized extremity osteosarcoma: combined results and prognostic factors from three European Osteosarcoma Intergroup randomized controlled trials. Ann Oncol. 2012; 23:1607- 1616

Telangiectatic osteosarcoma

25. Matsuno T, Unni KK, McLeod RA et al. Telangiectatic osteogenic sarcoma. Cancer. 1976 Dec;38(6):2538-47.

26. Mervak TR, Unni KK, Pritchard DJ et al. Telangiectatic osteosarcoma. Clin Orthop Relat Res. 1991 Sep;(270):135-9.

27. Murphey MD, wan Jaovisidha S, Temple HT et al. Telangiectatic osteosarcoma: radiologic-pathologic comparison. Radiology. 2003 Nov;229(2):545-53.

28. Weiss A, Khoury JD, Hoffer FA et al. Telangiectatic osteosarcoma: The St. Jude Children's Research Hospital's experience. Cancer. 2007 Apr 15;109(8):1627-37.

Small cell osteosarcoma

29. Sim F H, Unni K K, Beabout J W et al Osteosarcoma with small cells simulating Ewing's tumor. J Bone Joint Surg Am. 1979; 61:207-215.

30. Nakajima H, Sim F H, Bond J R et al Small cell osteosarcoma of bone: review of 72 cases. Cancer. 1997; 79:2095-2106.

31. Machado I, Alberghini M, Giner F et al Histopathological characterization of small cell osteosarcoma with immunohistochemistry and molecular genetic support: a study of 10 cases. Histopathology. 2010; 57:162-167.

Mangement of chemotherapy for osteosarcoma

32. Raymond A K, Ayala A G. Specimen management after osteosarcoma chemotherapy. Contemp Issues Surg Pathol. 1988; 11:157-181.

Intraosseous well differentiated osteosarcoma

33. Unni K K, Dahlin D C, McLeod R A et al Intraosseous well-differentiated osteosarcoma. Cancer. 1977; 40:1337–1347.

34. Kurt A M, Unni K K, McLeod R A. Low-grade intraosseous osteosarcoma. Cancer. 1990 Mar 15;65(6):1418-28.

Parosteal.osteosarcoma

35. Unni K K, Inwards C Y. Parosteal osteosarcoma. In: Dahlin's Bone tumors: general aspects and data on 10,165 cases. Sixth edition. Lippincott Williams & Wilkins, Philadelphia. 1994:158-168.
36. Okada K, Frassica F J, Sim F H et al. Parosteal osteosarcoma: a clinicopathological study. J Bone Joint Surg Am. 1994; 76:366-378
37. Wold L E, Unni K K, Beabout J W et al Dedifferentiated parosteal osteosarcoma. J Bone Joint Surg Am. 1984; 66:53-59.
38. Bertoni F, Bacchini P, Staals E L et al. Dedifferentiated parosteal osteosarcoma: the experience of the Rizzoli Institute. Cancer. 2005; 103:2373-2382.

Periosteal osteosarcoma

39. Unni K K, Dahlin D C, Beabout J W. Periosteal osteogenic sarcoma. Cancer. 1976; 37:2476-2485
40. Cesari M, Alberghini M, Vanel D et al. Periosteal osteosarcoma: a single-institution experience. Cancer. 2011; 117:1731-1735.
41. Grimer R J, Bielack S, Flege S et al Periosteal osteosarcoma--a European review of outcome. Eur J Cancer. 2005 Dec;41(18):2806-11.
42. Rose P S, Dickey I D, Wenger D E etal. Periosteal osteosarcoma: long-term outcome and risk of late recurrence. Clin Orthop Relat Res. 2006 Dec; 453:314-7.

High-grade surface osteosarcoma

43. Wold L E, Unni K K, Beabout J W et al High-grade surface osteosarcomas. Am J Surg Pathol. 1984; 8:181-186.
44. Okada K, Unni K K, Swee R G et al High grade surface osteosarcoma: a clinicopathologic study of 46 cases. Cancer. 1999; 85:1044-1054.
45. Staals E L, Bacchini P, Bertoni F. High-grade surface osteosarcoma: a review of 25 cases from the Rizzoli Institute. Cancer. 2008; 112:1592-1599.

Chapter *4: Malignant round cell tumors*

Ewing's sarcoma

Ewing's sarcoma is a primary malignant small round cell tumor of bone which always expresses CD 99, MIC 2 gene product. It characteristically shows t(11; 27)(q24, q12) translocation which results in the formation of the fusion gene EWSR1- FLI1. The term Primitive Neuroectodermal Tumor (PNET) is used synonymously.

Clinical findings

Ewing's sarcoma is a tumor of children and adolescents. More than 75 % of the tumors occur in the first two decades. However, it is uncommon in children below 5-year age. There is slight male predominance. Almost any bone in the body may be involved but 60 % occur in the lower extremities and pelvic girdle bones. Less frequently ribs, vertebrae, sacrum, skull bones and bones of hands and feet may be affected. The tumor presents with pain and bone expansion. There may be warmth and tenderness of the involved bone. The tumor can masquerade as acute osteomyelitis clinically, radiologically and even grossly.

Radiology

Radiologically, Ewing's sarcoma produces permeative lytic destructive lesion in long stretch of bone not unlike that seen in lymphomas or acute osteomyelitis. When the tumor destroys the cortex and extends in to extra-osseous region, there is lifting of the periosteum which results in characteristic onion-peel like reactive ossification (Fig. 4.1 A, B). There is varying degree of bone expansion with involvement of the surrounding soft tissues.

Grossly, the tumor appears greyish white, soft, friable and necrotic (Fig. 4.1 C). Often it may show liquefactive necrosis resulting in pus-like consistency further emphasizing its likeness to acute osteomyelitis.

Microscopic

Histologically, this is a highly cellular small round cell tumor with areas of necrosis. The small, blue, round cell tumors comprise a diverse group of malignant neoplasms in both children and adults. The tumors most commonly included in the differential diagnosis included Ewing's sarcoma/primitive neuroectodermal tumor (ES/PNET), neuroblastoma, rhabdomyosarcoma, poorly differentiated synovial sarcoma, lymphoblastic lymphoma, esthesioneuroblastoma, desmoplastic round cell tumor, mesenchymal chondrosarcoma, and blastemal predominant Wilms' tumor [1]. These tumors may be histologically indistinguishable, particularly when poorly differentiated or the cells are small, round to oval with vesicular nuclei and inconspicuous nucleoli. Mitotic activity may not be striking. The Ewing's tumor needs to be differentiated from a variety of small round "blue" cell tumors [2,3]. Some tumors are composed of large and more pleomorphic cells exhibiting prominent nucleoli; this is the large cell variant or atypical Ewing's tumor. This may be mistaken for large cell lymphoma or undifferentiated bone neoplasm. The biological behavior is similar to that of conventional Ewing's tumor [4]. The tumor cells are arranged in large sheets with fibrous bands of varying thickness separating them in compartments (Fig. 4.1 D, E). True rosettes, may or may not be seen.

The diagnosis of Ewing sarcoma with demonstration of CD 99[5,6] by immunohistochemistry in every case of Ewing sarcoma is recommended (Fig. 4.1 F). However, CD99 is not specific as other small round cell tumors namely; lymphoblastic lymphoma, mesenchymal chondrosarcoma, and small cell osteosarcoma may also express CD99. In such cases, fusion gene EWSR 1-FLI1 demonstration either by FISH (Fig 4.1 G) or by reverse transcriptase technique becomes necessary. This fusion gene occurs in more than 90% of cases [1].

Once a lethal tumor, the prognosis of Ewing sarcoma has vastly improved with the advent of newer chemotherapy protocols. Treatment of Ewing sarcoma is mainly chemotherapy with or without adjunct surgery and radiation. Five-year survival is now expected to be almost 70 % [7].

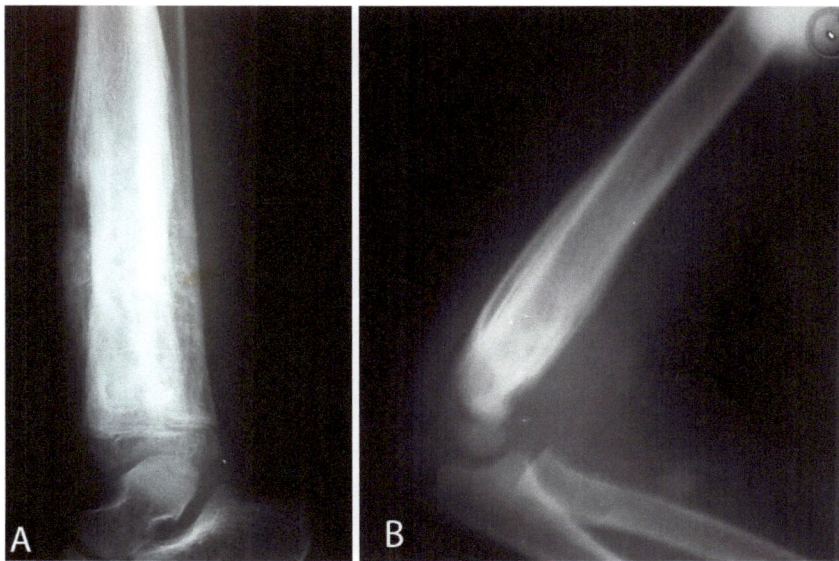

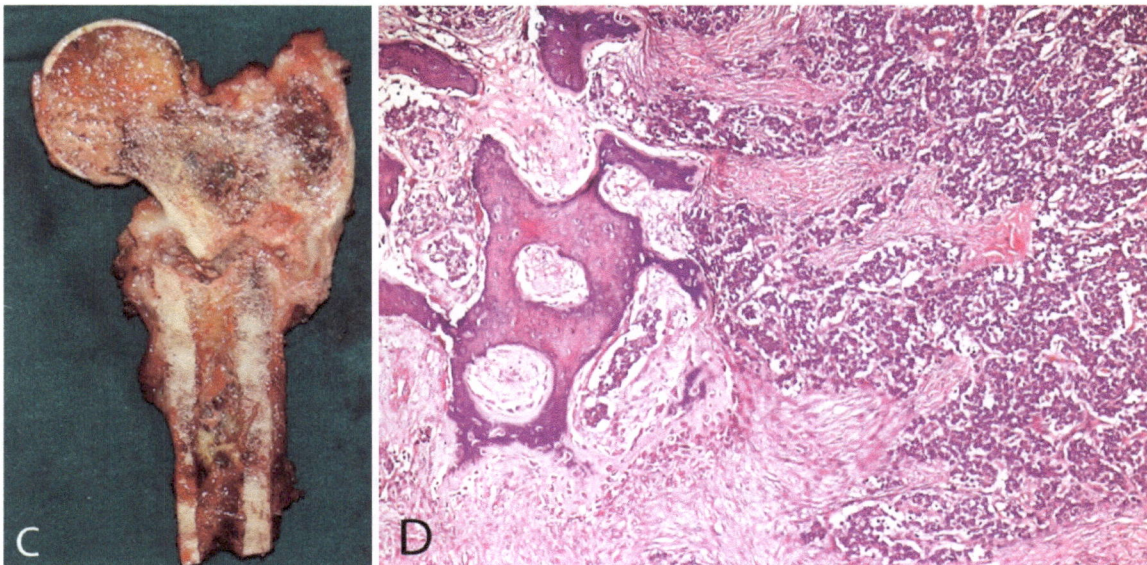

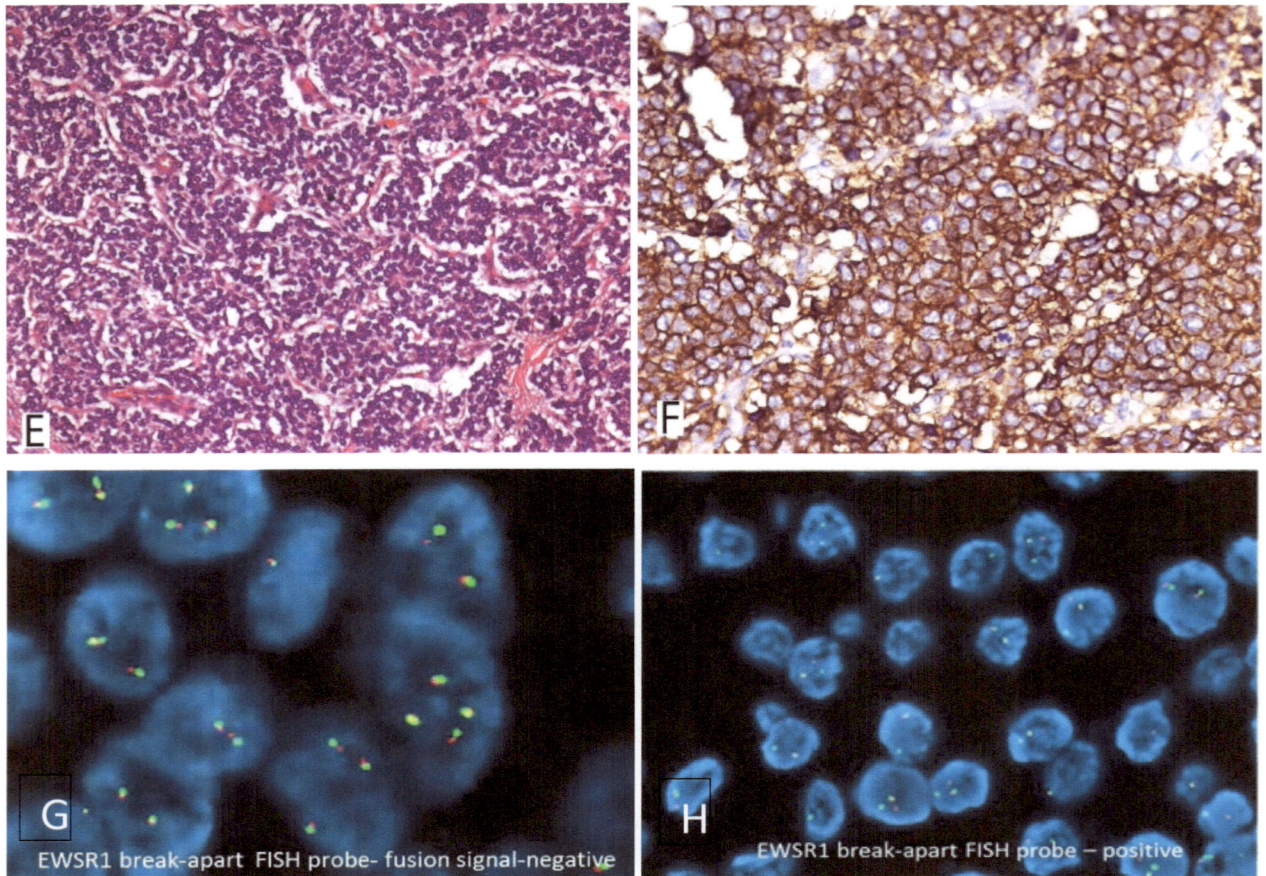

Fig. 4.1 (A, B) Ewing sarcoma: destructive, permeative lesion in the lower end of tibia with multi-layered periosteal reactive new bone formation, the "onion peel" appearance; (C) upper end of femur with pathological fracture; (D) necrosis and marked bone destruction are seen; (E) high power view of the tumor; (F) CD99 antibody immunostaining: prominent membrane positivity of all tumor cells (G) EWSR1 break-apart FISH probe – negative, (H) EWSR1 break-apart FISH probe – Positive

Primary Malignant Lymphoma

Primary bone lymphoma (PBL) is a group of rare lymphoid malignancies, and is defined as a lymphoma that is confined to the bone or bone marrow without evidence of a systemic disease at the time of diagnosis and initial staging [8]. This tumor is a distinct entity and distinction from disseminated lymphoma is clinically significant because primary bone lymphoma has better prognosis. This tumor usually affects adults. Radiologically these present as infiltrative sclerotic/ lytic lesions (Fig. 4.2 A, B).

Once the possibility of lymphoma is suspected, immunohistochemistry confirms the diagnosis and assists in the immunophenotypic classification. The bulk of primary bone lymphomas are B cell lymphomas, most commonly diffuse large B cell lymphoma (Fig. 4.2 C, D). It is important to know that lymphoblastic lymphoma may be positive for CD99 and negative for CD45, an immunoprofile that overlaps with that of Ewing sarcoma [9]. Application of lymphoma panel for immunohistochemistry will readily make the lymphoma diagnosis, including classification.

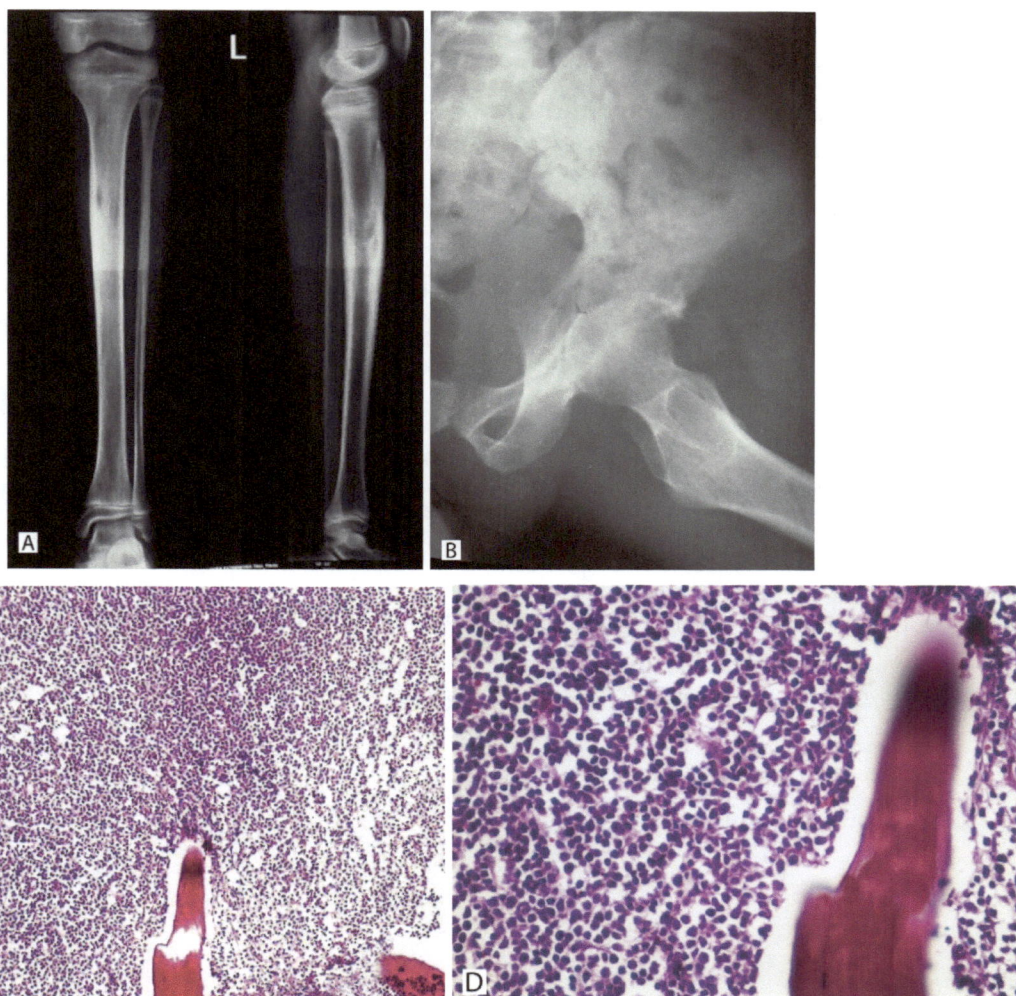

Fig. 4.2 Malignant lymphoma: (A) permeative sclerotic lesion with fuzzy borders in tibia and (B) permeative densely sclerotic lesion in the ilium; (C) crush artefact is a characteristic feature; (D) close up view of lymphoma shows a monotonous population of neoplastic lymphoid cells

References for Chapter 4

Ewing sarcoma

1.   Folpe AL, Hill CE, Parham DM, et al. Immunohistochemical Detection of FLI-1 Protein Expression A Study of 132 Round Cell Tumors With Emphasis on CD99-Positive Mimics of Ewing's Sarcoma/Primitive Neuroectodermal Tumor Am J Surg Pathol 2000; 24: 1657–1662

2.   Hameed M: Small round cell tumors of bone. Arch Pathol Lab Med 2007; 131:192-204.

3.   Machado I, Noguera R, Mateos E A et al. 2011 The many faces of atypical Ewing's sarcoma: a true entity mimicking sarcomas, carcinomas and lymphomas. Virchows Arch 458: 281-290

4.   Nascimento AG, Unni K K, Pritchard D J et al 1980 A clinicopathologic study of 20 cases of large cell (atypical) Ewing's sarcoma of bone. Am J Surg Pathol 4: 29-36

5. Weidner N, Tjoe J 1994 Immunohistochemical profile of monoclonal antibody O13: antibody that recognizes glycoprotein p30/32MIC2 and is useful in diagnosing Ewing's sarcoma and peripheral neuroepithelioma. Am J Surg Pathol 18: 486-4945.

6. Stevenson AJ, Chatten J, Bertoni F et al CD99 (p30/32MIC2) neuroectodermal/Ewing's sarcoma antigen as an immunohistochemical marker: review of more than 600 tumors and the literature experience Appl Immunohistochem 1994 2: 231-240

7. Granowetter L, Womer R, Devidas M, et al. Dose-intensified compared with standard chemotherapy for non-metastatic Ewing sarcoma family of tumors: a Children's Oncology Group Study J Clin Pathology 2009; 27:2536-2541

Malignant lymphoma

8. Bhagavathi S, Micale MA, Les K, et al. Primary Bone Diffuse Large B-cell Lymphoma Clinicopathologic Study of 21 Cases and Review of Literature Am J Surg Pathol 2009; 33:1463–1469)

9. Ozdemirli M, Fanburg-Smith JC, Hartmann DP, et al. Precursor B-Lymphoblastic Lymphoma Presenting as a Solitary Bone Tumor and Mimicking Ewing's Sarcoma: A Report of Four Cases and Review of the Literature Am J Surg Pathol 1998 22:795-804

Chapter 5: Fibroblastic tumors

Metaphyseal fibrous defect /Non ossifying fibroma

Metaphyseal fibrous defect is not a neoplasm, but a degenerative disorder of growing bone. This is a lesion of young, and many disappear spontaneously as the bone matures.

Clinical findings

Majority occur in long tubular bones, mainly lower end of femur, and upper end of tibia. Humerus, radius, ulna are less commonly involved. Rarely rib, clavicle may be affected. In long tubular bones, metaphysis is the commonest site; rarely diaphysis may be involved.

The lesion remains asymptomatic or may be detected incidentally. Rarely local pain may be complained of. Uncommonly, the lesion may present with pathological fracture.

Radiologically[1,] the lesion is typically in the cortex, being lucent and well defined with sclerotic borders. The inner surface may be trabeculated and scalloped (Fig. 5.1 A).

Gross appearance of the curetted material is greyish white, granular, firm with brownish or yellowish areas.

Microscopic

The lesion is composed of spindle shaped fibroblasts, arranged in loose sheets, fascicles and in storiform pattern with scattered small multinucleated osteoclastic giant cells. There may be sprinkling of lymphocytes, and occasional clumps of foamy macrophages (xanthoma cells). There may be deposits of hemosiderin pigment in the stroma (Fig. 5.1 B, C D). The lesion closely resembles benign fibrous histiocytoma. Many pathologists and radiologists use the term interchangeably, though incorrectly. Benign fibrous histiocytomas grow to larger size and are more cellular and compact; while metaphyseal fibrous defects are essentially degenerative, and the fibrous spindle cells are arranged loosely; and degenerative changes like foamy macrophages and hemosiderin pigment deposits are seen more frequently (Fig. 5.1 D, E, F)

Many lesions remain asymptomatic for years; and some even disappear as the bone matures. If symptomatic, a confident diagnosis can be made radiologically and the lesion need not be excised. However, if the diagnosis is in doubt, or if there is impending fracture, the lesion may be curetted and cemented. This treatment is curative.

Metaphyseal fibrous defect is a solitary lesion in majority of the cases. However, in rare cases multiple lesions may be seen.

Jaffe – Campanacci syndrome[2] has multiple lesions of metaphyseal fibrous defect associated with skin pigmentation, and other extraskeletal abnormalities. Recently there has been suggestion that Jaffe-Campanacci syndrome is indeed part, of forme fruste of Neurofibromatosis type 1.

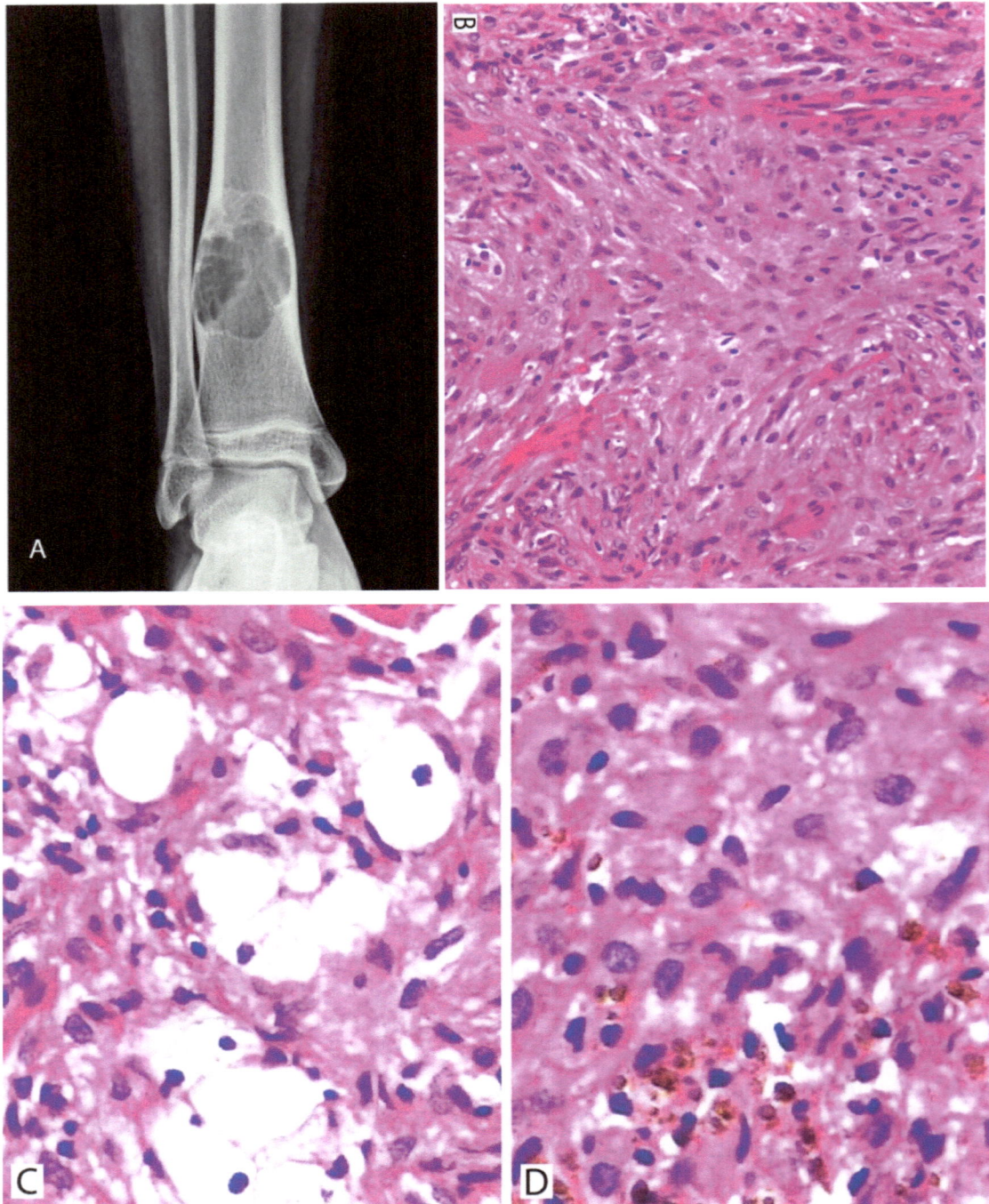

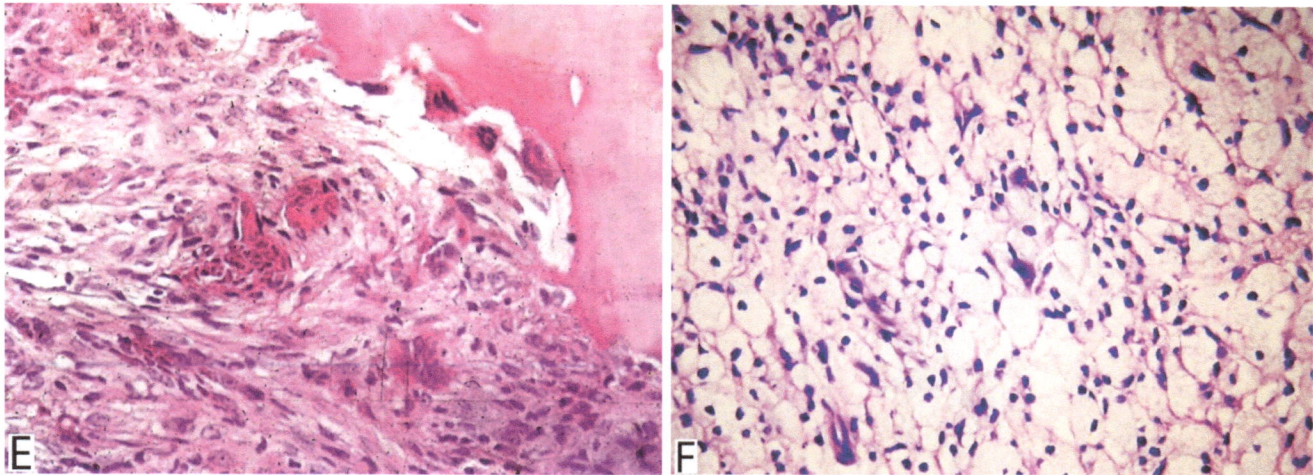

Fig. 5.1 A Case of metaphyseal fibrous defect: (A) large lobulated lucent lesion with sharply defined scalloped borders, lower metaphysis of tibia.; (B) benign spindle lesion with storiform pattern; (C) clusters of foamy macrophages; (D) hemosiderin pigment deposits in lower 1/3rd.(E) A small (few millimeter) osteolytic lesion incidentally detected on x-ray, note osteoclastic giant cells eroding the host bone trabeculum and sheets of fibroblasts and few histiocytes; (F) sheets of foamy histiocytes

Desmoplastic fibroma

Desmoplastic fibroma is a rare primary bone tumor, histologically resembling desmoid-type fibromatosis of soft tissues. These occur mainly in adults and radiologically present as slowly growing lytic destructive metaphyseal lesion in long tubular bones. Radiological differential diagnoses include other lytic lesions such as aneurysmal bone cyst, giant cell tumor, chondromyxoid fibroma, and low-grade fibrosarcoma[3]. Grossly, it is a well circumscribed, firm and whitish tumor (Fig.5.2 A, B). Histological diagnosis is easy with no variation in its morphology. It is typically hypocellular with abundant stromal collagenization. Mitotic figures are hard to find (Fig. 5.2 C, D)[4]. The differential diagnosis includes fibrous dysplasia and low grade osteosarcoma. Parosteal osteosarcoma and low-grade central osteosarcoma are two types of low-grade osteosarcomas that show similar clinical behaviors, histological features, and genetic background (i.e., amplified sequences of 12q13-15, including MDM2 and CDK4). Low-grade osteosarcoma is often confused with benign lesions, and ancillary techniques to enhance diagnostic accuracy are necessary. MDM2 and CDK4 immunostains reliably distinguish low-grade osteosarcoma from benign histological mimics, and their combination may serve as a useful adjunct in this difficult differential diagnosis.[5]. The tumor is locally aggressive with a high rate of recurrence. Recurrence following curettage or en block resection is 72% and 17% respectively [6].

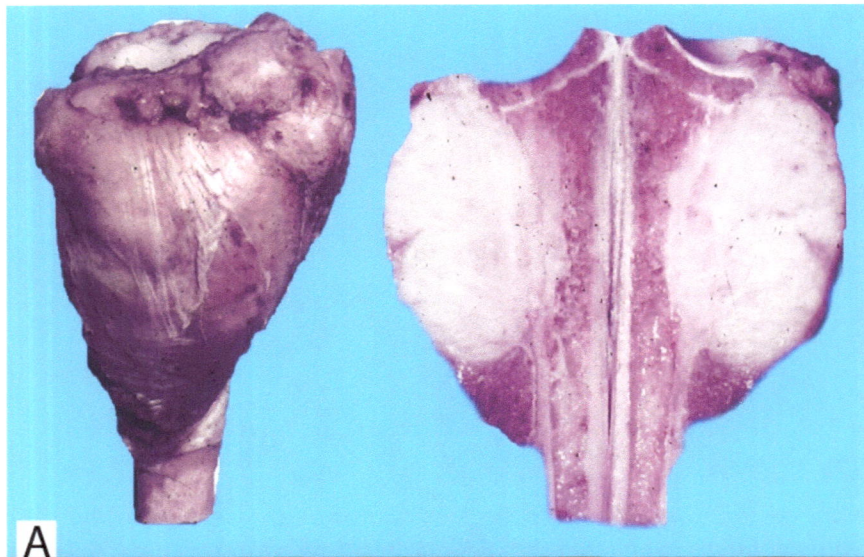

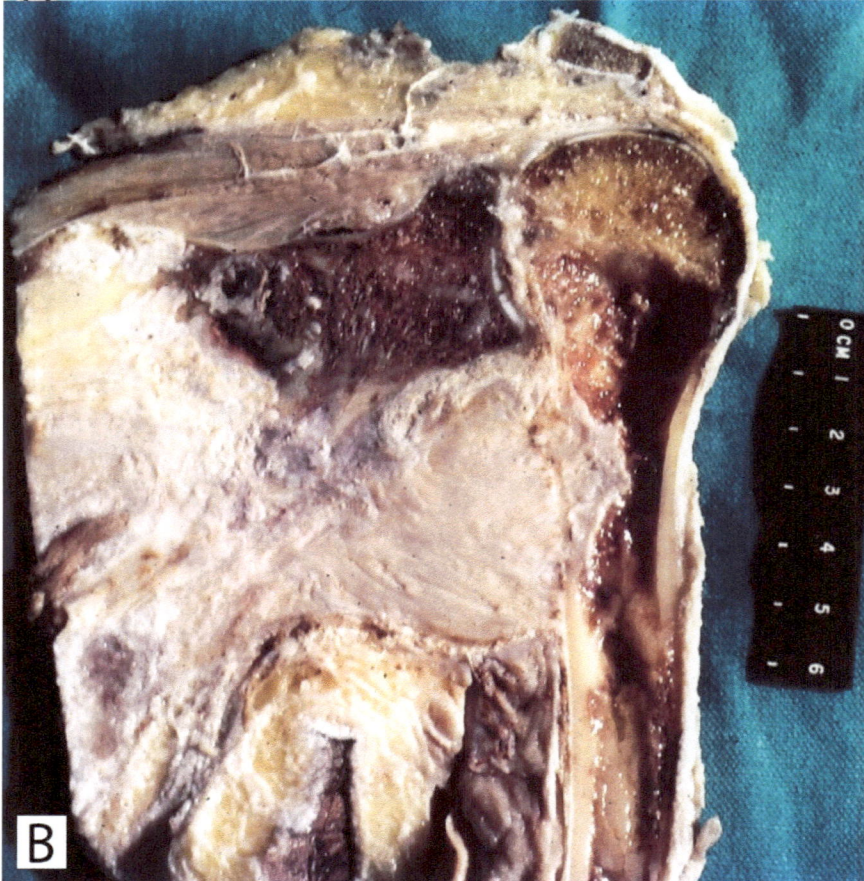

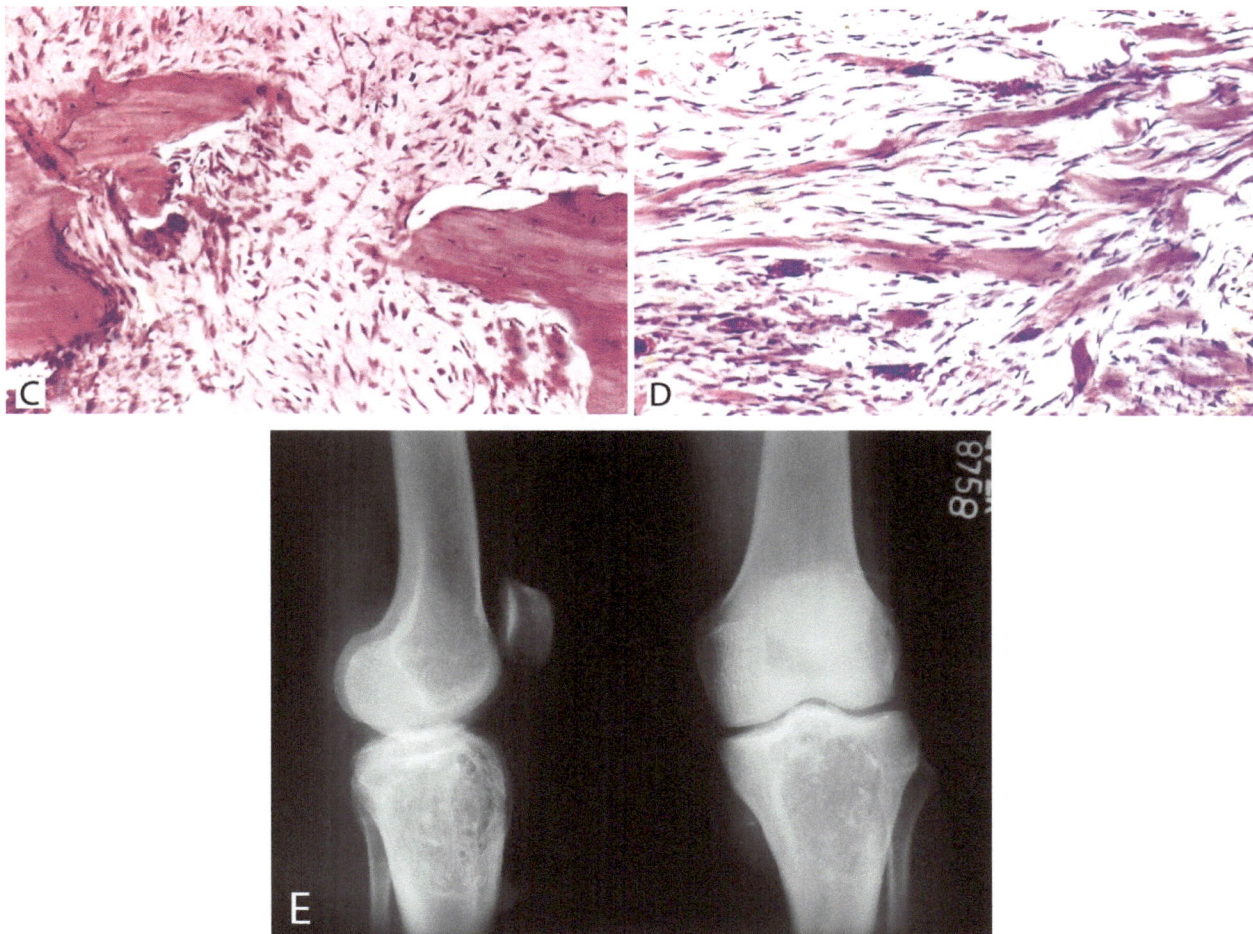

Fig. 5.2 Desmoplastic fibroma: (A) resected upper end of fibula bearing a circumscribed firm white tumor invading the cortex; (B) a very large whitish tumor invading the cortex and medulla of the humerus, it has filled and enlarged the axilla; three previous excisions of a recurring desmoplastic fibroma and finally the upper limb was fixed and completely immobile; (C) edematous fibroblastic tissue infiltrating and destroying a trabeculum; (D) this desmoplastic fibroma involving humerus and axilla shows keloid like histological picture; (E) a lytic circumscribed lesion with a well-defined border; this is from another case.

Fibrosarcoma It is a rare bone tumor and occurs in elderly subjects with location typically in metaphysis with extension to epiphysis or diaphysis. Well differentiated fibrosarcomas have well defined margins and high grade tumors radiologically present as any other destructive bone sarcoma with extensive lytic changes (Fig. 5.3 A, B). Grossly the tumor is homogenous, whitish and firm (Fig. 5.3 C). Histologically, it is similar to those occurring in the soft tissues. Differentiation from the fibroblastic variant of osteosarcoma may be difficult (Fig. 5.3 D), particularly in needle biopsy specimens. Fibrosarcoma has been reported in association with a number of conditions: prior radiation therapy, Paget's disease of bone, giant cell tumor, osteochondroma, fibrous dysplasia, bone infarcts, chronic osteomyelitis etc.[7]. Most fibrosarcomas tend to be well differentiated with broad fascicles of spindle shaped fibroblasts with a richly collagenous focal hyalinized matrix. The diagnosis of poorly differentiated (Fig 5.3 D) or pleomorphic fibrosarcomas is difficult, even after immunohistochemical and ultrastructural studies [8]. Fibroblast is an inert cell with no diagnostic morphologic attributes.

The 10 year survival was 83% in low grade and 34% in high grade fibrosarcoma, in one series [8].

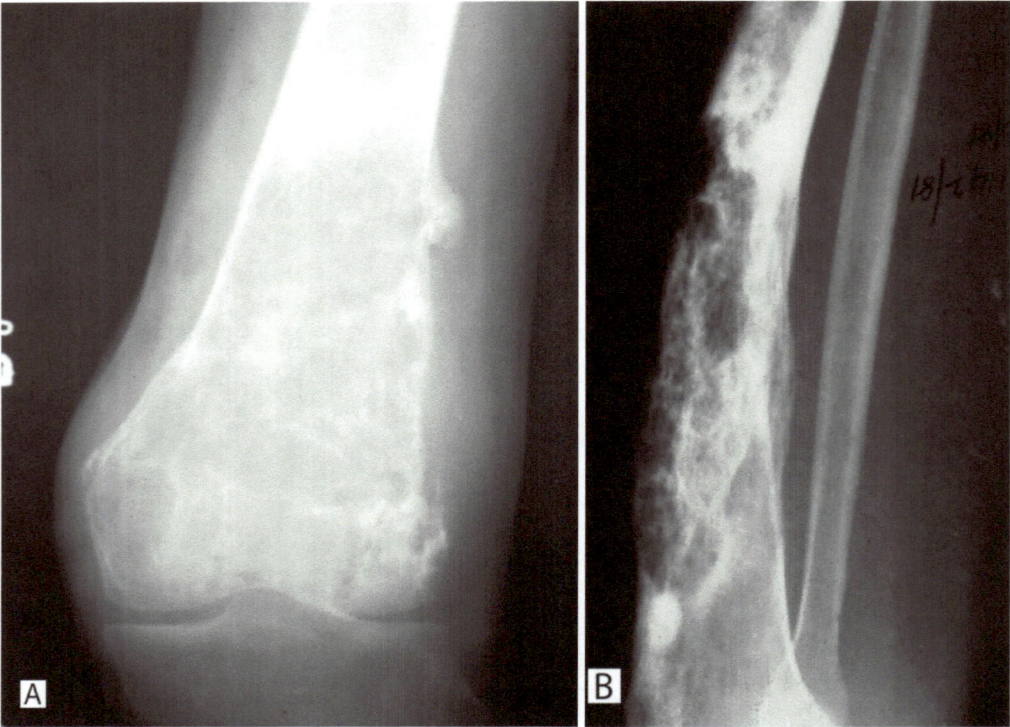

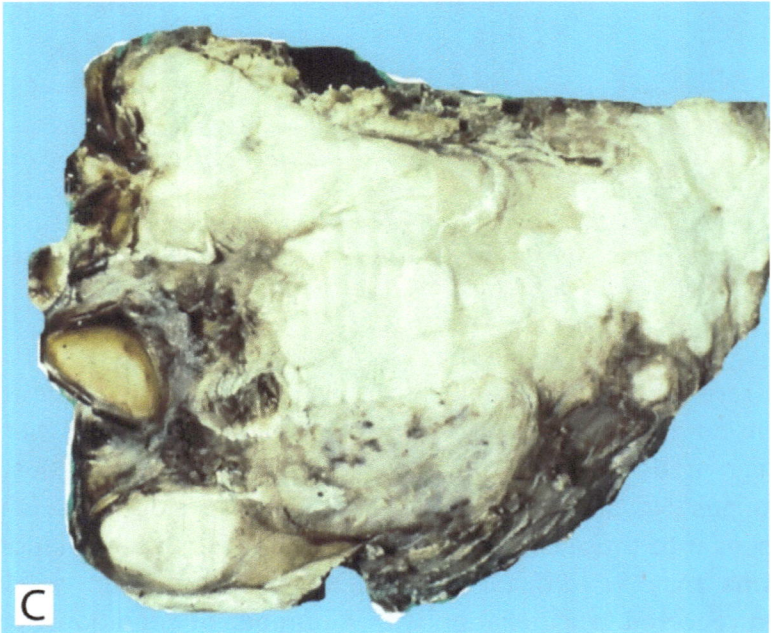

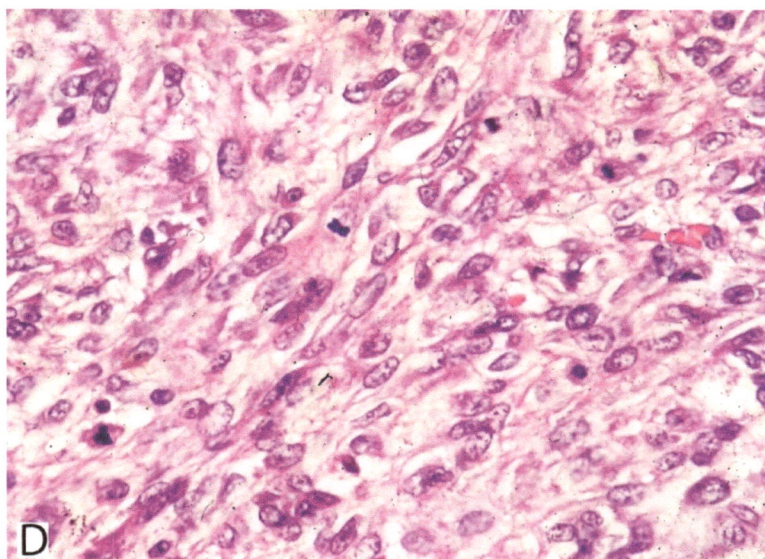

Fig. 5.3 Fibrosarcoma: (A) extensive lytic destructive tumor involving metaphysis and extending to epiphysis of lower femur; (B) a large ragged lytic destructive lesion in metaphysis of lower tibia; (C) a homogenous whitish tumor diffusely involving the scapula; (D) a high grade spindle cell fibrosarcoma of scapula

Undifferentiated high grade pleomorphic sarcoma (Malignant fibrous histiocytoma)

Definition

Undifferentiated high grade pleomorphic sarcoma (Malignant fibrous histiocytoma) is a primary pleomorphic sarcoma of bone with a variable morphology in which the tumor cells do not produce osteoid or cartilage matrix. This definition has been in vogue for 40 years, until the WHO classification of soft tissue tumors was published in the year 2002. What has been termed MFH by surgical pathologists over a period of four decades has been replaced by the term undifferentiated pleomorphic sarcoma, which is the most common pattern among 5 different histological types of MFH. This paradigm change had its origin in the publication on search for a correct histogenesis of the tumor Undifferentiated high grade pleomorphic sarcoma (Malignant fibrous histiocytoma), the question: is histiocyte a cell of origin for this tumor?

Fletcher et al [9] reassessed 159 tumors initially diagnosed as pleomorphic sarcomas morphologically, immunohistochemically and ultrastructurally. Only 13% of the cases were eligible for consideration as MFH but these tumors did not show evidence of histiocyte/macrophage differentiation. To ascertain whether MFH tumor cells actually express the features of histiocytes like monocyte/macrophage lineage, antigenic and enzymatic studies were carried out in 13 cases of MFH of different histological subtypes [9]. It was proved that MFH tumor cells do not express the enzyme profile of cells of monocyte/macrophage lineage. The author concluded that MFHs are primitive mesenchymal neoplasms, most likely poorly differentiated fibroblasts and are unrelated to true histiocytic neoplasms.

Antonescu and others [10] carried out a comparative ultrastructural study of primary fibrosarcoma (4 cases) and Undifferentiated high grade pleomorphic sarcoma (Malignant fibrous histiocytoma) (8 cases) of bone to look for evidence of a spectrum of fibroblastic differentiation. In conclusion, fibroblastic differentiation and collagen production was noted in all cases. The findings support the hypothesis that the fibroblast and its variants are the predominant cell types found in these tumors, suggesting that the diagnostic entity MFH should be reclassified as a pleomorphic fibrosarcoma.

A few bone tumors have been still diagnosed as Undifferentiated high grade pleomorphic sarcoma (Malignant fibrous histiocytoma) for want of any better label. MFH have been reported in long tubular bones, mainly in adult patients. Radiologically, the tumor presents as bone destructive lesions with no characteristic radiological features (Fig.5.4 A). Histologically, MFH of bone are similar to its soft tissue counterpart (Fig. 5.4 B, C).

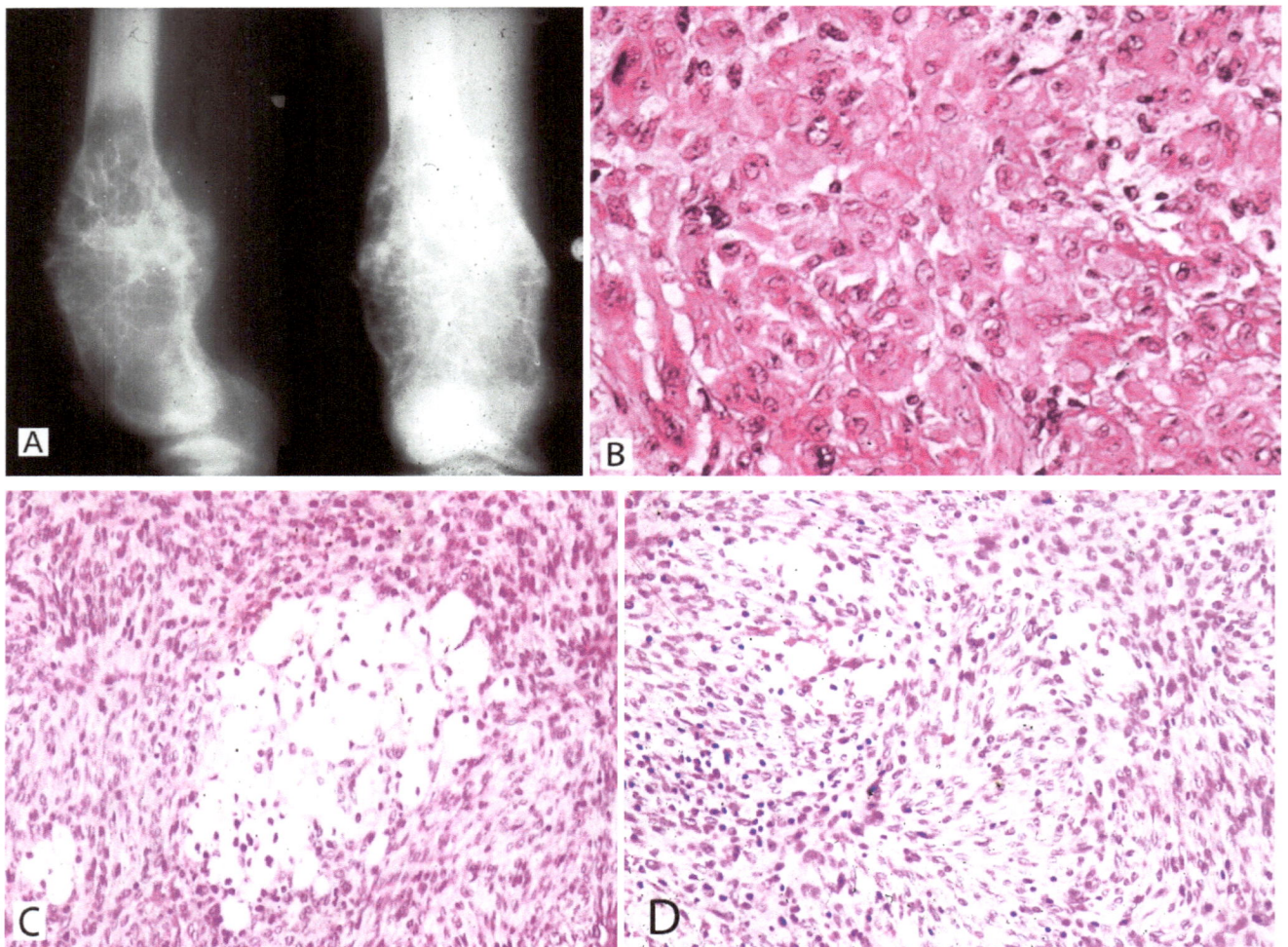

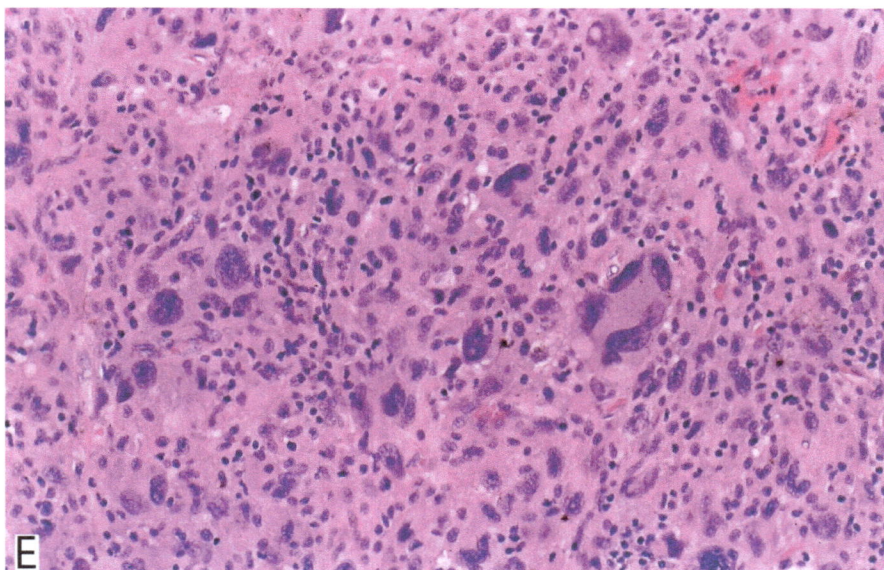

Fig. 5.4 (A) Large destructive tumor involving metaphysis and diaphysis; (B) sheets of medium size cells exhibiting acidophilic cytoplasm and mild to moderate nuclear anaplasia; (C) sheets of lipid containing histiocytes in the center and surrounding spindle cell component; on the basis of this picture alone the diagnosis will be benign fibrous histiocytoma; D) spindle cell component with storiform pattern, occasional mitosis seen; E) this picture is of another case showing a pleomorphic undifferentiated malignant tumor with large number of bizarre tumor giant cells, this represents the most anaplastic variety of MFH (old terminology)

The term MFH is not yet totally abandoned and survives because of its familiarity, popularity and usage for almost half a century. At this point the authors would keep the term MFH for convenience.
In a series of 90 cases11 of MFH of bone the overall survival rates were 34% at 5 years, and 28% at 10 years. Surgery alone did not appear to be successful (5-year survival, 28%). Adjuvant chemotherapy improved the survival rate only in patients who underwent adequate surgery (5-year survival, 57%).

Huvos reported an overall survival of 71% and 53% at 2 years and 5 years respectively in a series of 130 cases[12.] Of skeletal fibrosarcoma. He observed important prognostic factors were age of the patient and whether tumor was primary de novo or secondary sarcoma. Older patients and those with secondary sarcoma did substantially worst. In a clinico-pathological evaluation of 81 cases[13], seventy-eight percent of the lesions arose *de novo* and 22% in preexisting conditions (secondary sarcoma). Histologically, most of the tumors were classified as the storiform pleomorphic type, although other histologic subtypes were identified. The prognosis depended on the types of surgical margins involved. Patients with wide or radical margins had a better prognosis than patients in whom the margins were contaminated. Some patients who received radiation therapy alone became long term survivors.

References for Chapter 5

Metaphyseal fibrous cortical defect (Non-ossifying fibroma)

1.   Jeep WH, Choe BY, Kang HS et al (1998) Non-ossifying fibroma: characteristics at MR imaging with pathologic correlation. Radiology 2009; 1:197–202

2.   Mankin HJ, Trahan CA, Fondren G, Mankin CJ Non-ossifying fibroma, fibrous cortical defect and Jaffe-Campanacci syndrome: a biologic and clinical review. Chir Organi Mov. 2009 May; 93(1):1-7.

Desmoplastic fibroma

3.   Gebhardt MC, Campbell CJ, Schiller AL, Mankin HJ: Desmoplastic fibroma of bone. A report of eight cases and review of the literature J Bone Joint Surg Am 1985; 67:732-47
4.   Inwards C Y, Unni K K, Beabout J W et al. 1991 Desmoplastic fibroma of bone. Cancer 68: 1978-1983
5.   Yoshida A, Ushiko T, Motoi T, et al. Immunohistochemical analysis of MDM2 and CDK4 distinguishes low-grade osteosarcoma from benign mimics. Mod Pathol 2010; 23:1279-88.
6.   Green M, Sirikumara M Desmoplastic fibroma of mandible Ann Plast Surg 1987; 19: 284-290

Fibrosarcoma

7.   Kahn LP, Vigorita V Fibrosarcoma of Bone in Pathology & Genetics: Tumors of soft tissue and bone, WHO classification of tumors (Ed: Fletcher CDM, Unnikrishnan K K, Mertens F) Page 289 IARC Press Lyon 2002
8.   Bertoni F. Campannacci R, Calderon P, et al Primary central (medullary) fibrosarcoma of Bone Semin Diagn Pathol 1984; 1:185-198

Undifferentiated high grade pleomorphic sarcoma (Malignant fibrous histiocytoma)

9.   Fletcher CDM. Pleomorphic Undifferentiated high grade pleomorphic sarcoma (Malignant fibrous histiocytoma) : Fact or Fiction?. Am J Surg Pathol 1992; 16:213-218
10. Antonescu C R, Erlandson R A, Huvos A G Primary fibrosarcoma and Undifferentiated high grade pleomorphic sarcoma (Malignant fibrous histiocytoma) of bone: a comparative ultrastructural study—evidence of a spectrum of fibroblastic differentiation. Ultrastruct Pathol 2000 ; 24: 83-91
11. Capannacci R, Bertoni F, Bacchini P et al. Undifferentiated high grade pleomorphic sarcoma (Malignant fibrous histiocytoma) of bone: the experience at the Rizzoli Institute: report of 90 cases. Cancer1984; 54: 177-187
12. Huvos AG, Heilweil M, Bretsky S S The pathology of Undifferentiated high grade pleomorphic sarcoma (Malignant fibrous histiocytoma) of bone: a study of 130 patients Am J Surg Pathol 1985;9: 853-871
13. Nishida J, Sim F H, Wenger D E et al. Undifferentiated high grade pleomorphic sarcoma (Malignant fibrous histiocytoma) of bone: a clinicopathologic study of 81 patients. Cancer 1997; 79: 482-493

Chapter 6: Vasoformative tumors

Epithelioid hemangioma

Hemangiomas are much more common in soft tissues and include capillary, cavernous, epithelioid, histoid, and sclerosing histological patterns. Only the epithelioid hemangioma of bone is discussed here. The clinical and pathologic features of 50 epithelioid hemangiomas of bone were analyzed by Nielsen et al [1]. Epithelioid hemangioma (EH), previously designated as angiolymphoid hyperplasia with eosinophilia is a well-recognized distinct clinicopathologic entity. Epithelioid hemangioma of bone is not an uncommon tumor and is one of a group of vascular neoplasms that also include epithelioid hemangioendothelioma and epithelioid angiosarcoma and these are characterized by plump epithelioid endothelial cells. Epithelioid hemangiomas of bone are often mistaken for low grade hemangioendothelioma or angiosarcoma [2]. Many hemangiomas of bone remain asymptomatic and hence diagnosed on routine X rays done for some other purpose. Majority of skeletal lesions are solitary, involving the long bones, but up to 25% are multifocal, usually restricted to a regional location. In the Nielson series of 50 cases 40% occurred in long tubular bones, 18% in the distal lower extremity, 18% flat bones, 16% vertebrae, and 8% small bones of the hands. The tumor consists of well-formed capillaries and few solid capillaries, all lined by endothelial cells with acidophilic cytoplasm and plump nuclei (Fig. 6.1 A, B). Follow-up information revealed that 4 patients experienced a local recurrence; and 1 patient developed limited involvement of a regional lymph node. Epithelioid hemangioma is successfully treated with curettage or marginal en bloc excision

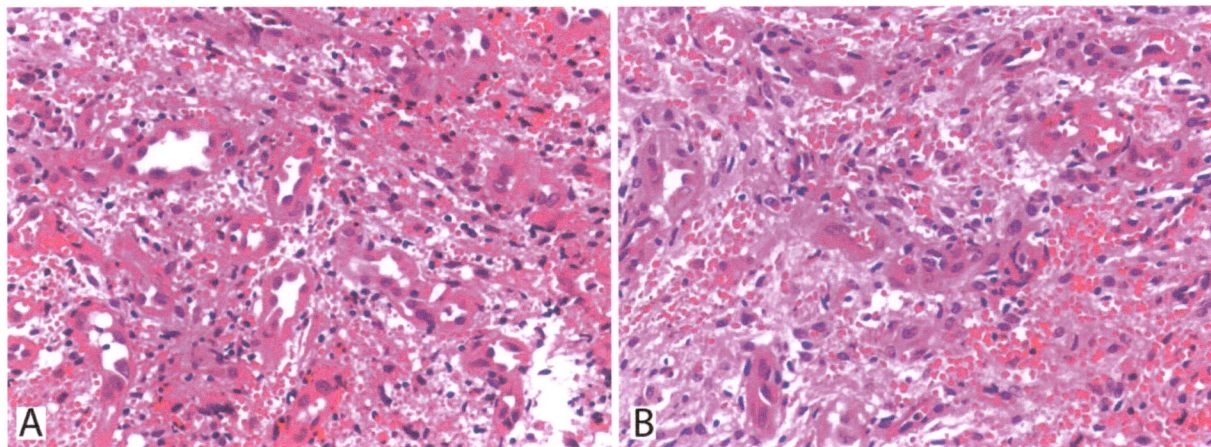

*Fig. 6.1 Epithelioid hemangioma (A) well-formed capillaries and plump lining endothelial cells; B) in this illustration the capillaries the capillaries appear solid with no nuclear atypia, **or** mitosis.*

Epithelioid Hemangioendothelioma

The term hemangioendothelioma is used to indicate a vascular tumor with intermediate grade of malignancy. It is a tumor of endothelial origin; biologically, it is a low-grade malignancy with a clinical course between that of a hemangioma and a conventional angiosarcoma. Often the term is used with no specific meaning except that the endothelial cells are plump and prominent. Clinically, the only symptom may be local tenderness or pain, particularly when the lesion involves a superficial bone. There is no specific x-ray finding and the most common feature is the presence of purely lytic lesion without periosteal reaction. Histologically, a few well-formed vessels and some narrow irregular vessels, all lined by large plump coarsely hyperchromatic nuclei, are present (Fig. 6.2 A) in some parts this tumor is solid with no vessels seen (Fig. 38 B). No mitosis or necrosis is present, however. Keer et al reported a series of 40 cases of this tumor from Mayo Clinic[3]. More than 50% (22 of 40 cases) of the tumors were multicentric, with a predilection for femur and tibia (60%). Hemangioendotheliomas rarely occur in other sights like liver and bone. It was not possible to predict the outcome on the basis of histological findings; visceral involvement was the most important criterion to predict prognosis. Surgical resection is treatment of choice; radiotherapy may be useful for inaccessible tumors.

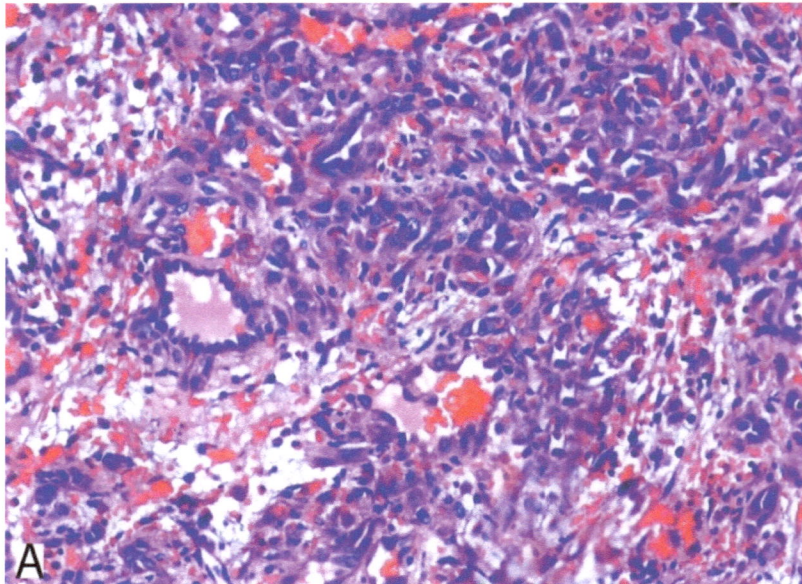

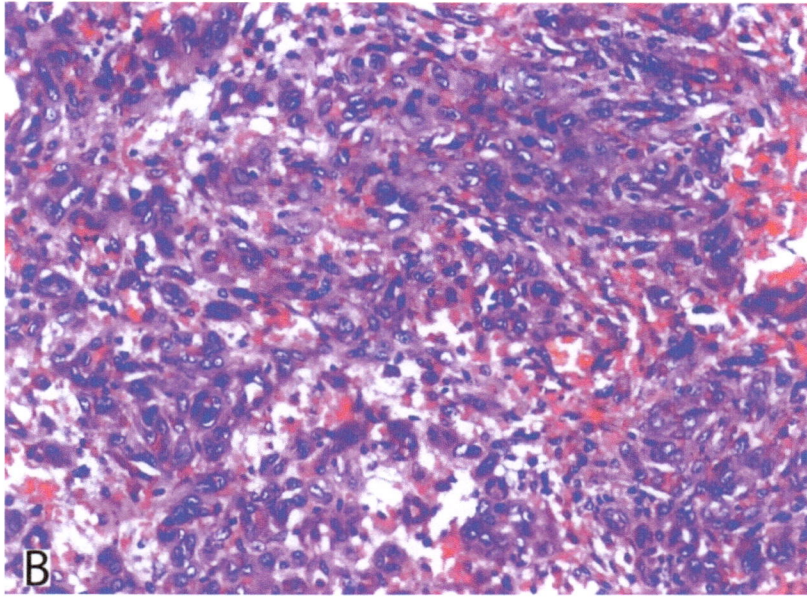

Fig. 6.2 Hemangioendothelioma: (A) well-formed vessels and capillary buds, large hyperchromatic endothelial nuclei and hypercellularity; (B) a solid cellular pattern, and quite prominent nuclei but no mitotic activity or necrosis seen

Angiosarcoma

The terminology of malignant vascular tumors has been controversial. The current practice is to use the term hemangioendothelioma for low grade vascular tumor and angiosarcoma for high grade vascular tumor. There may still be some debate but the term angiosarcoma for high grade tumor is widely accepted. Angiosarcoma of bone is uncommon with no distinctive radiological features. Histologically, the tumor has the same morphology as that of soft tissue counterpart. A bewildering number of histological manifestations have been described. The patterns include: features similar to capillary or cavernous hemangioma, Dabska tumor, spindle or epithelioid hemangioendothelioma and carcinoma. 70% of cases display epithelioid cells that are arranged in nests, clusters, papillae, and gaping vascular channels[4]. Angiosarcoma may be multicentric and behave in an aggressive manner. In particular, epithelioid angiosarcoma can, frequently metastasize, and results in death in a short clinical course. Verbeke et al described distinct histological features in 42 cases of primary angiosarcoma of bone and found that majority show keratin positivity and pathologist should avoid mistaking it for carcinoma [5]. Histologically angiosarcoma needs to be distinguished from metastatic carcinoma (Fig. 6.3 A, B, D). Immunohistochemistry with CD 31 or CD34 antibody is of great help in establishing endothelial nature of the tumor (Fig. 6.3 C). In the illustrated case, the diagnosis was metastatic adenocarcinoma on H & E stain alone. The cells are clearly epithelial with acidophilic cytoplasm with hyperchromatic nuclei, and gland formation.

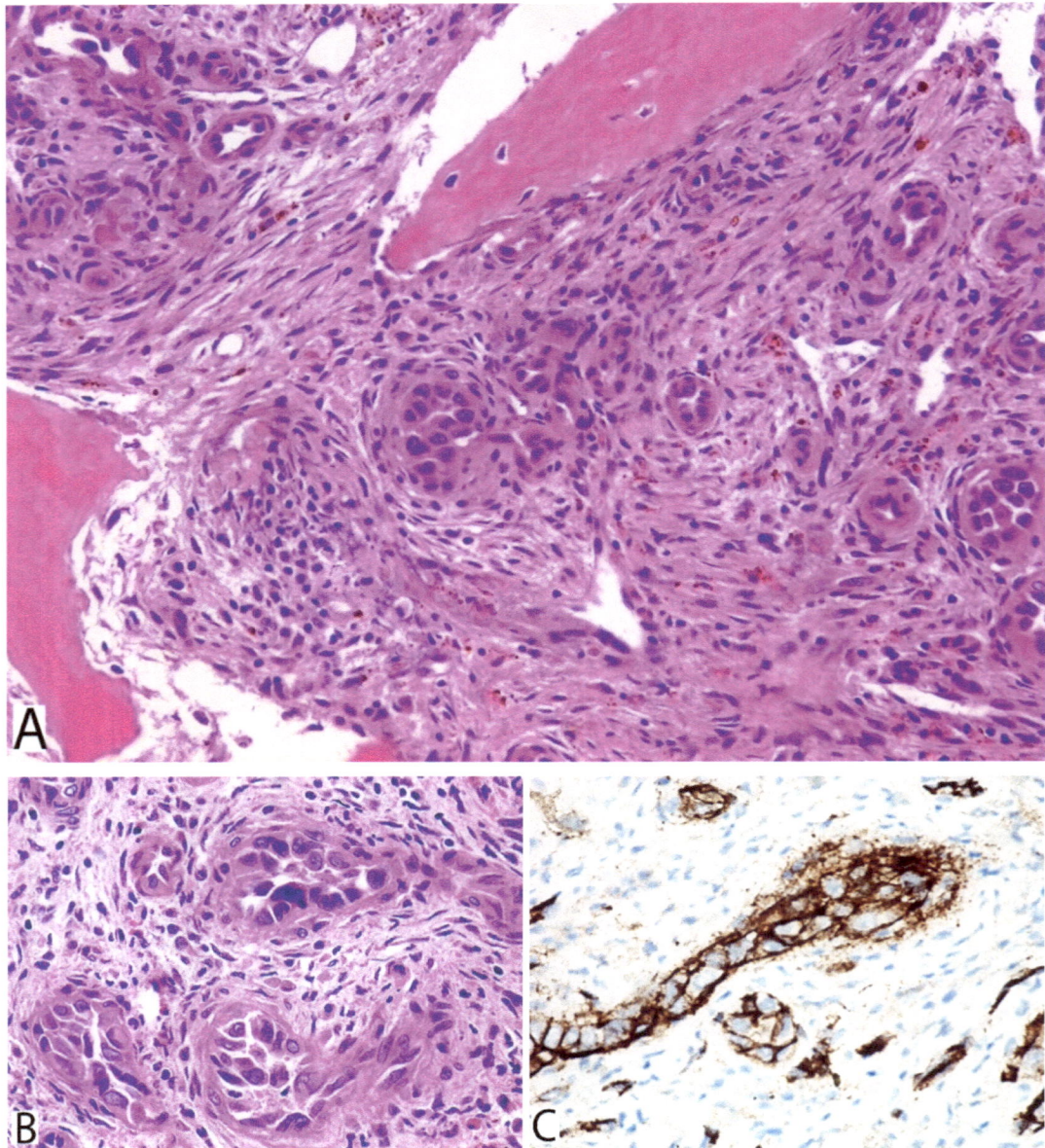

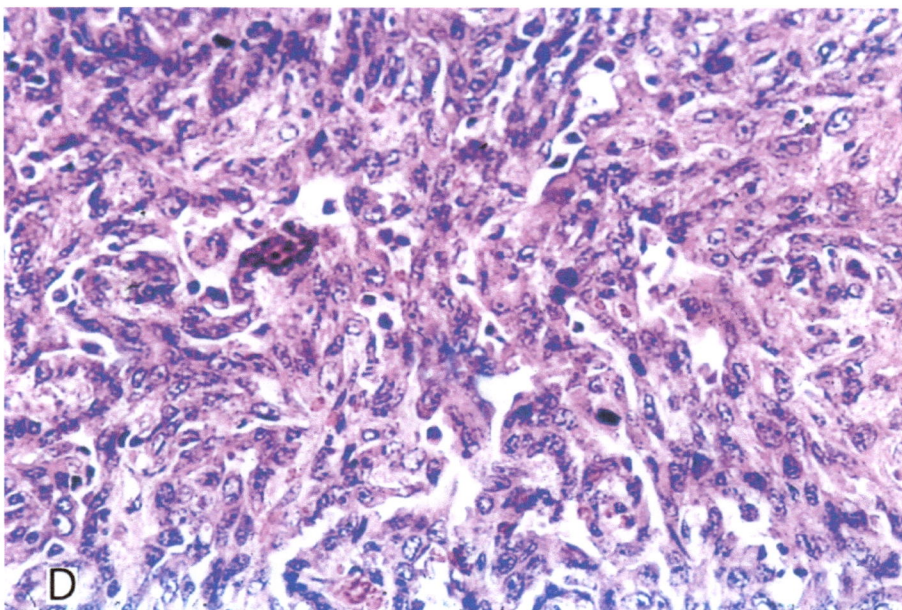

Fig.6.3 angiosarcoma: (A) many thick vessels lined by strongly hyperchromatic nuclei, note bland bone trabeculae; (B) close up of neoplastic vessels showing prominent nuclear anaplasia; (C) endothelial cells display strong membrane staining with CD 34 antibody; (D) high power view of a solid cellular angiosarcoma with many bizarre abnormal mitoses, picture from another case, adenocarcinoma was ruled out with IHC.

These tumors can be multifocal, frequently metastasize, and result in the patient's death in a short clinical course. It is important to distinguish them from other epithelioid vascular tumors and metastatic carcinoma because of the differences in their management and clinical outcome[6].

References for Chapter 6

Epithelioid hemangioma

1. Nielson GP, Shrivastav K, Kattapurum S, et al. Epithelioid hemangioma of bone revisited: a study of 50 cases. Am J Surg Pathol 2009; 33:270-277
2. O'Connell JX, Kattanpuram S, Mankin HS, et al Epithelioid hemangioma of bone. A tumor often mistaken for low grade malignant hemangioendothelioma or angiosarcoma Am J Surg Pathol 1993; 17:610-617

Hemangioendothelioma

3. Kleer C G, Unni K, McLeod R A 1996 Epithelioid hemangioendothelioma of bone. Am J Surg Pathol 20: 1301-1311

Angiosarcoma

4. Meis-Kindblom J M, Kindblom L G 1998 Angiosarcoma of soft tissue: a study of 80 cases. Am J Surg Pathol 22: 683-697

5. Verbeke SL, Bertoni F, Bacchini P, Sciot R, Fletcher CD, Kroon HM, Hogendoorn PC, Bovée JV. Distinct histological features characterize primary angiosarcoma of bone. Histopathology. 2011 an;58(2):254-64.
6. Deshpande V, Rosenberg A E, O'Connell J X et al. 2003 Epithelioid angiosarcoma of the bone: a series of 10 cases. Am J Surg Pathol 27: 709-716

Chapter 7: Giant cell tumor (GCT) of bone

Definition

The GCT typically occurs in epiphysis or rarely in metaphysis of long bones and consists of compact sheets of non-fibrogenic spindly cells with intimately mixed large osteoclastic giant cells. GCT is often locally aggressive but very rarely develops a sarcomatous transformation.

Clinical features

GCT is usually seen in age group 20 to 40 years and presents with pain and swelling at the ends of long bones. The majority of cases involve lower end of femur, upper end of tibia, proximal humerus and distal radius. Involvement exclusively of epiphysis is the diagnostic "sine qua non" of GCT and authors find that this is the most useful feature in the differential diagnosis of giant cell containing lesions.

Radiology

Plain x-ray of the lesion in long bones typically shows an expanding large eccentric radiolucency in the epiphysis (see panel 7.0). In a Mayo clinic series of 1682 GCTs, only 14 cases (0.83%) were accepted as truly non-epiphyseal (10 were metaphyseal and 4 diaphyseal) in location[1]. Chondroblastoma is the only other tumor that exclusively involves the epiphysis.

GCT of axial skeleton are uncommon and rather difficult to treat, due to the limited surgical accessibility and proximity to spinal cord and nerve roots. In a study of 282 cases of GCT, only 19 cases affected vertebral column (6 cases in spine, and 13 in sacrum). GCTs at these sites have high local recurrence rate and may present with neurological deficit[2].

GCT of bones of hand and foot

GCT of bones of hand and foot are uncommon and the prevalence of these tumors in several large series varied from 0.9% to 4% in hand and 1.2% to 2.4% in foot. The tumors at these sites have some peculiar features compared with GCT of long bones in that, they show female predominance, younger age, typical epimetaphyseal x ray features and more aggressive behavior[3].

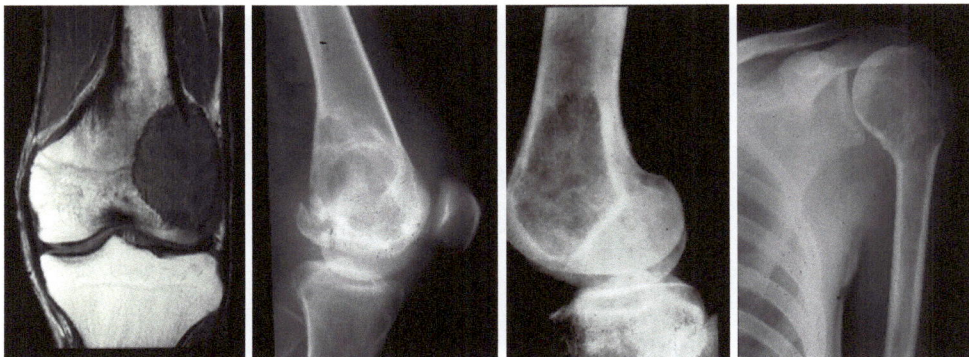

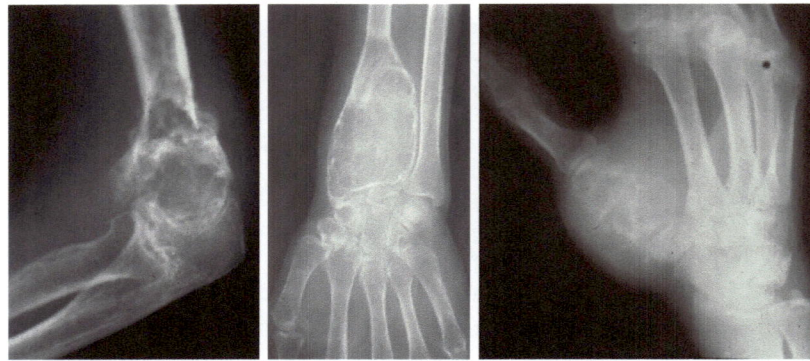

Fig.7.0 The panel shows epiphyseal or meta-epiphyseal osteolytic lesions in femur (MRI), recurrent tumor in lower end femur, femur (lower end), humerus (upper end), humerus recurrent tumor, radius (lower end) and 1st metacarpal respectively All images display GCT in epiphysis Note extension of epiphyseal lesion into metaphysis in many.

Gross

It is usually a large mass of soft reddish brown tissue and exactly corresponds to the radiological appearance in its eccentric location and fairly well defined area of bone destruction (Fig. 7.1 A). The lesion is well demarcated by a thin, often incomplete, shell of reactive bone. In a few cases, a cluster of blood filled spaces is encountered and this can mimic gross appearance of aneurysmal bone cyst, when extensive. Destruction of the cortex with extension to soft tissues is not uncommon.

Microscopic

The histological appearance is characteristic and almost monotonous. Dense sheets of uniform round to oval or elongated non-fibrogenic stromal (undefined mesenchymal) cells and uniformly interspersed large osteoclastic giant cells containing 50-100 nuclei are present (Fig.7.1 B, C). The nuclei of the stromal cells are identical to those of giant cells. In fact, experts are unanimous the truly neoplastic cells are the spindle stromal cells, and not the giant cells. Mitotic activity to the tune of 2 to 10 / 10 HPF may be present but atypical mitoses do not occur. The possibility of giant cell rich sarcoma may be entertained if atypical or particularly tripolar mitoses are present. Many retrogressive or reparative changes, namely old hemorrhage, sheets of foamy histiocytes, hemosiderin deposits, cystic degeneration and fibrosis are commonly encountered.

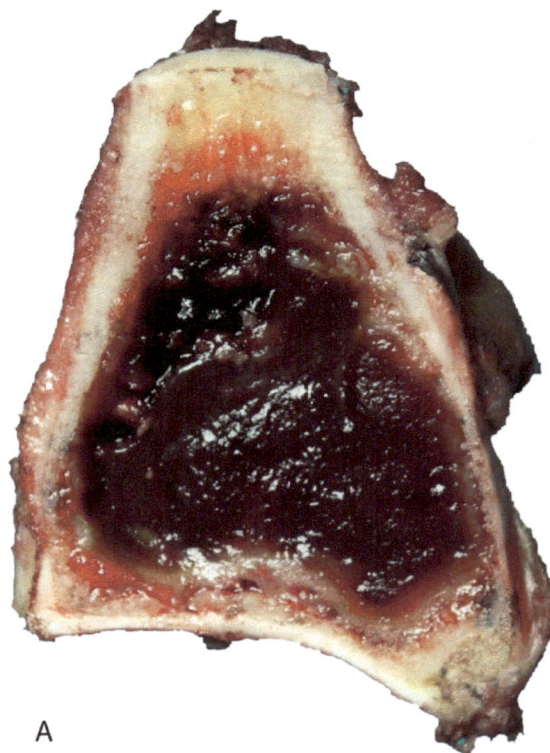

A

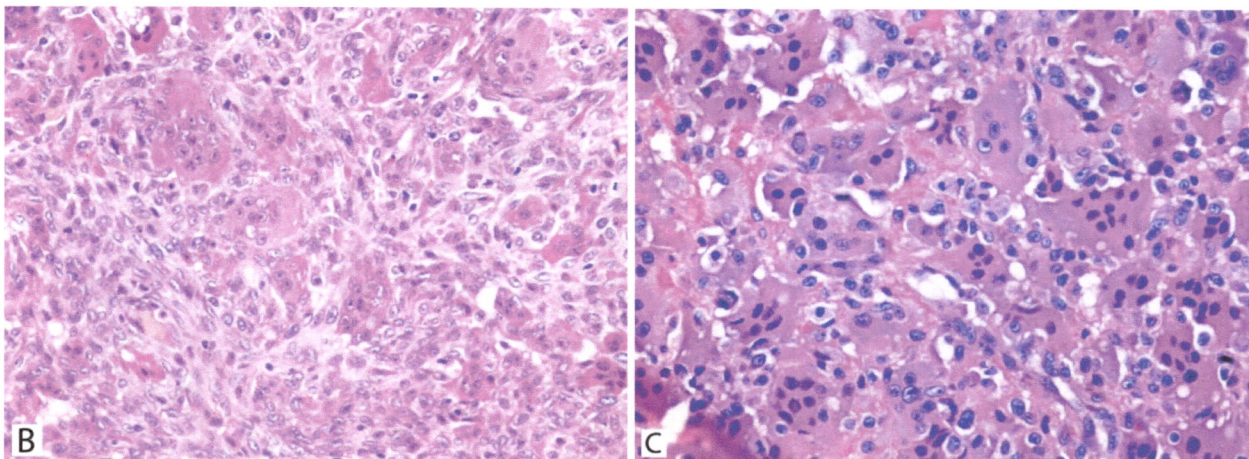

B

C

Fig.7.1 (A) upper end of tibia showing a well-defined hemorrhagic tumor with intact cortex and clear margins; (B,C) both photographs show similar typical structure of GCT, note that the nuclei of stromal cells are identical to those of osteoclasts.

Biological Behavior of Giant cell tumor of bone

GCT is potentially a locally aggressive tumor. The behavior of giant cell tumor has been regarded with suspicion and apprehension since its recognition. The concept of malignancy, when one discusses GCT of bone, has not been well defined. Even after study of many large series, the prediction of biological behavior, i.e., grading of these tumors has remained controversial. The subject is presented under the following:

1) Recurrence of GCT with consistent benign histological picture

The tumor is inherently locally invasive and frequent episodes of recurrences are not uncommon. In the case illustrated here, GCT had three recurrences over a 6-year period and finally destroyed the bone with extension to soft tissues (Fig. 7.2 A). After a block resection of proximal tibia with knee joint replacement patient remained disease free for further five years. At the third recurrence the excised tissue showed typical GCT with a totally benign morphology (Fig. 7.2 B) [4, 5, 6]

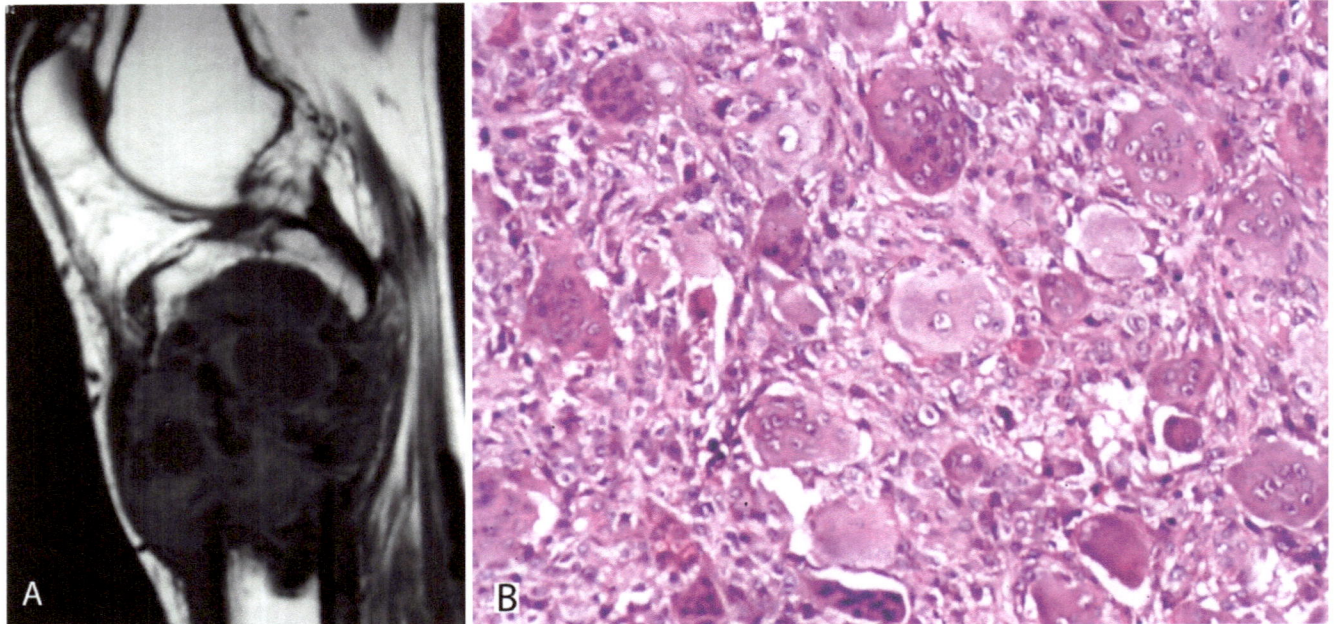

Fig.7.2 Aggressive GCT extending to soft tissues (A) upper end of tibia showing marked destruction and expansion with loss of cortex and involvement of soft tissues; (B) the photomicrograph presents a non-malignant morphology of GCT, even at the 3rd destructive recurrence.

2) GCT with histologically benign pulmonary metastasis

This is indeed an enigmatic phenomenon and has been reported in 42 out of a total of 1308 cases (3.2%) of benign GCT in one cumulative series'. In another large series of 649 cases (from single institution) of benign GCT of bone treated over a period of 22 years, 14 patients (2.1%) had lung metastases. The patients were treated with metastatectomy and all were alive at the end of 6 year follow up. Many studies have shown that none of the patients died owing to their metastatic disease regardless of whether they had metastatectomy or chemotherapy. It has been demonstrated that vascular invasion is seen outside the boundary of the GCT, when the tumor is vigorously curetted. This indicates mechanical transportation of the otherwise benign tumor cells to lung, lymph nodes or soft tissues ("metastases") This does not influence survival. And this is quite unlike metastases of transformed malignant cells[7].

3) Primary malignant GCT, ab initio

Primary malignant GCT (PMGCT) is a high grade sarcoma (Fig. 7.3), which should be seen side by side with unequivocal benign GCT. This is an extremely uncommon occurrence[8, 9].

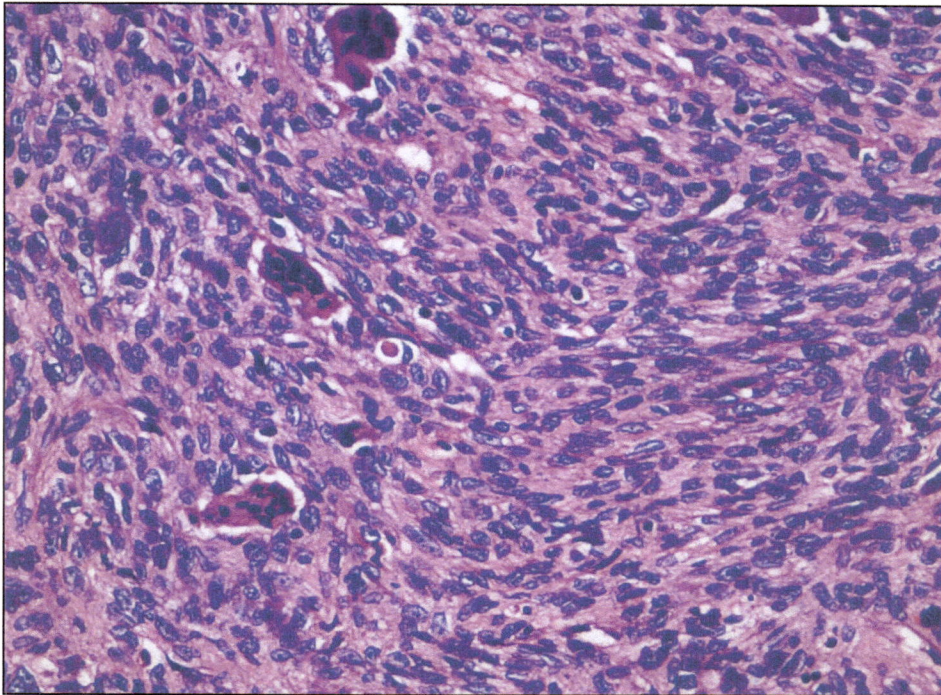

Fig. 7.3 Primary malignant GCT: Much of the tissue is occupied by typical spindle cell sarcoma, three residual osteoclasts are present; elsewhere areas of benign giant cell tumor were demonstrated

4) Secondary malignant GCT usually occurs years after radiation or surgery.

A known case of GCT, treated earlier, recurs as malignant tumor several years later at the same site (Fig. 7.4 A, B, C). Care should be taken to exclude giant cell rich osteosarcoma that was misdiagnosed as GCT initially, that has now recurred.

Malignant component in the recurrent tumor may be either fibrosarcoma or osteosarcoma.

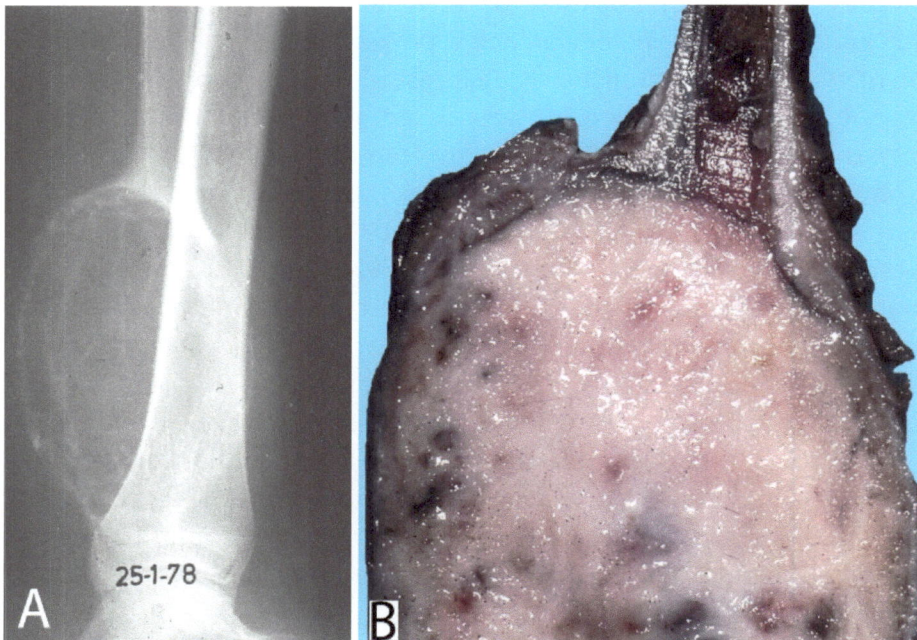

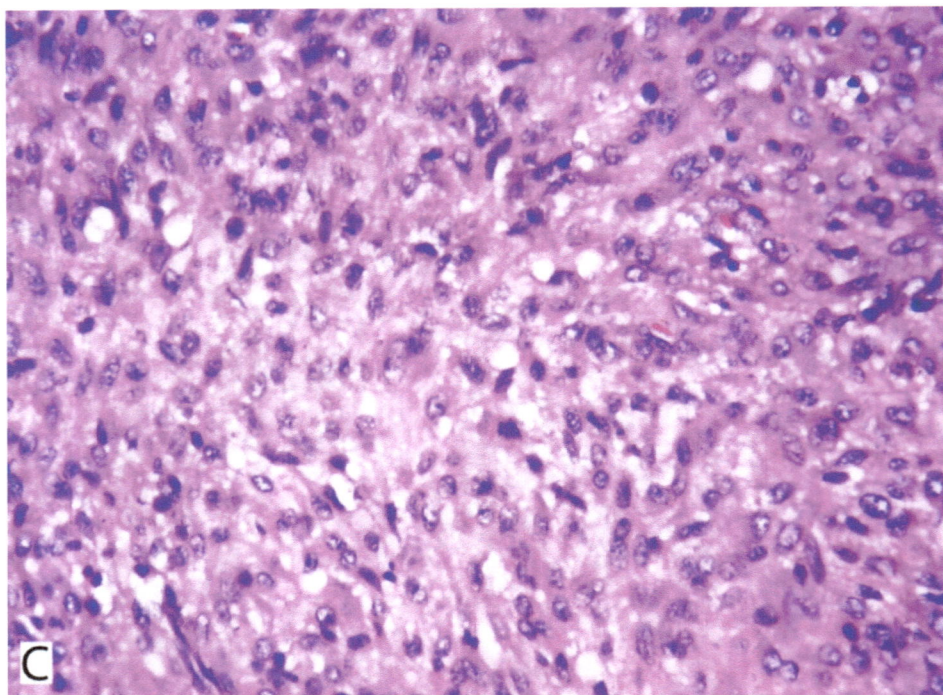

Fig. 7.4 Secondary malignant GCT: this patient had 10-year history of recurrent GCT, the last recurrence presented with a huge tumor mass above ankle joint: (A) X-ray of this large smooth osteolytic tumor at lower end of fibula; (B) gross appearance of resected tumor bearing fibula; (C) an actively mitotic spindle cell sarcoma with no residual GCT

Denosumab in the treatment of giant cell tumor of bone

The recent discovery of the role of Receptor Activator Nuclear factor kB (RANK) and RANK Ligand pathway in the pathogenesis of giant cell tumor has opened new and promising possibility in the treatment of this disease. As mentioned earlier, the stromal spindle cells are the true neoplastic cells of giant cell tumor of bone and have molecular and biologic features of osteoblasts. These neoplastic stromal mesenchymal cells characteristically express RANK L which regulates induction and proliferation of monocytes and formation of osteoclastic giant cells. These osteoclastic giant cells in turn result in the characteristic lytic expansile lesion seen on x ray picture. RANK / RANK L pathway regulates progression of the disease, and its metastatic potential. Suppression of RANK L results in reduced osteoclast formation and bone resorption, and enhances bone formation by the spindle stromal cells. Denosumab is human IgG 2 monoclonal antibody that binds soluble and membrane RANK L with high affinity, and effectively reduces osteoclast formation and tumor progression[10, 11.] Denosumab has now been approved by the FDA of USA for the treatment of giant cell tumor in cases where surgical alternative would result in unacceptable morbidity. Initial success of denosumab in halting the progression of the disease has resulted in increased use of this treatment modality, though long term effect is yet to be proved. Appropriate dosage and duration of treatment are yet to be assessed. Curetted tumor following treatment with Denosumab shows great reduction in number of osteoclasts or their complete absence with abundant osteoid formation in the stroma. A lytic spindle cell and giant cell predominant tumor is converted in to predominantly osteoblastic spindle cell tumor

(Fig. 7.5 A, B,C,D) This not only halts progression of the disease, but also aids in complete extirpation of the tumor surgically [12]

Thus, some studies have focused on histology as a measure of treatment response. Most significantly, denosumab treated GCT with abundant bone deposition may mimic GCT that has undergone malignant transformation. One recent publication on the subject compared histologically characterized treated GCTs with malignant neoplasms arising in GCTs. It was found that unlike the latter, denosumab treated GCTS showed less severe atypia, reduced mitotic activity, and lack of infiltrate growth pattern [13].

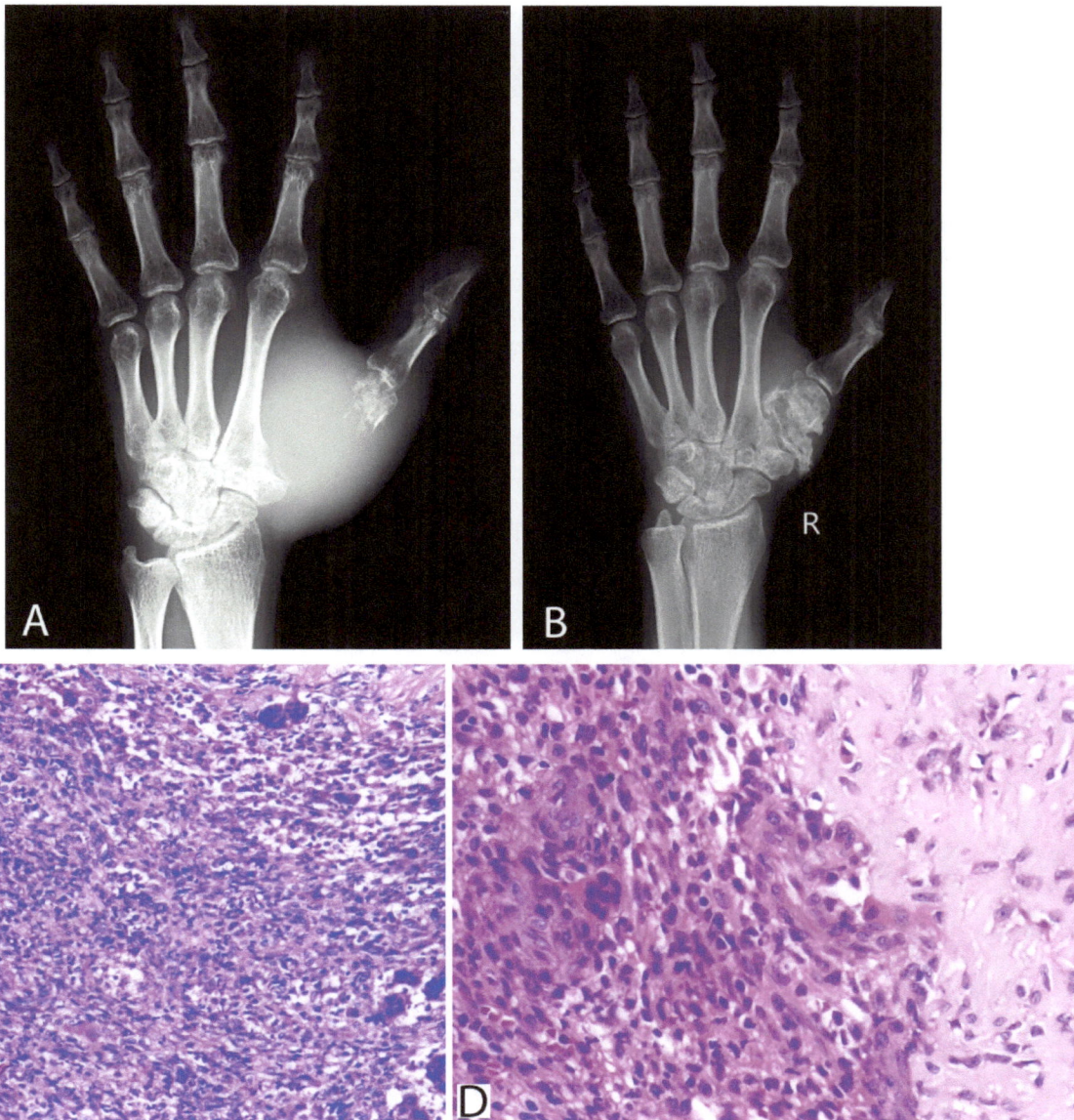

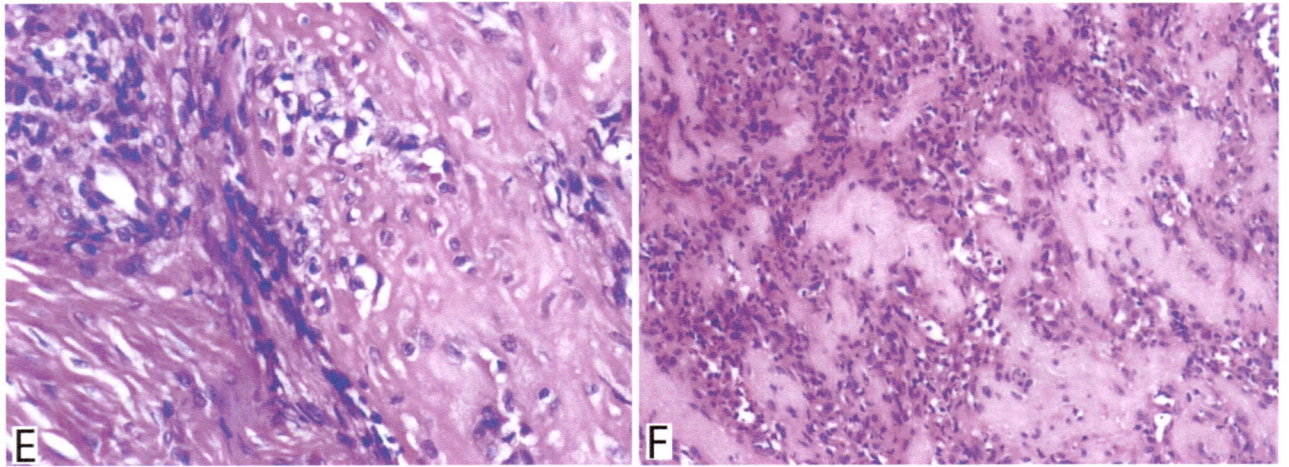

Fig. 7.5.(A) large destructive GCT involving right first metacarpal (B) post denosumab x-ray showing almost complete shrinking of the tumor and regular bone formation in the metacarpal bone (C) denosumab treatment leads to almost complete disappearance of osteoclasts with replacement by actively proliferating mesenchymal stromal cells (D) in this view only a single osteoclast has remained, note hyalinization with a vague appearance of osteoid (E) total loss of osteoclasts with replacement by mesenchymal stromal cells and fibroblastic tissue (F) many islands of osteoid separated by islands of stromal cells

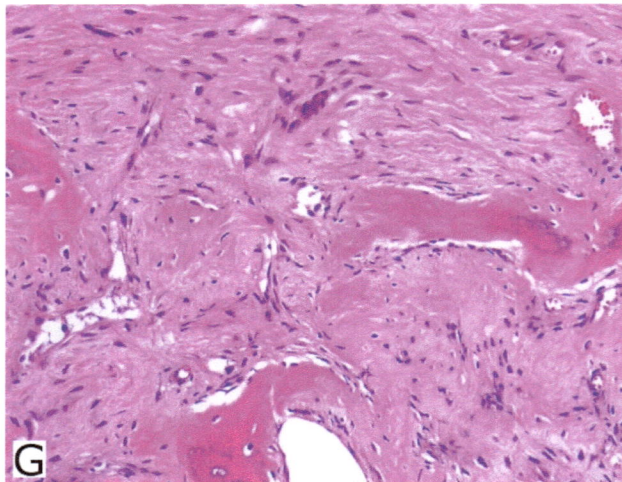

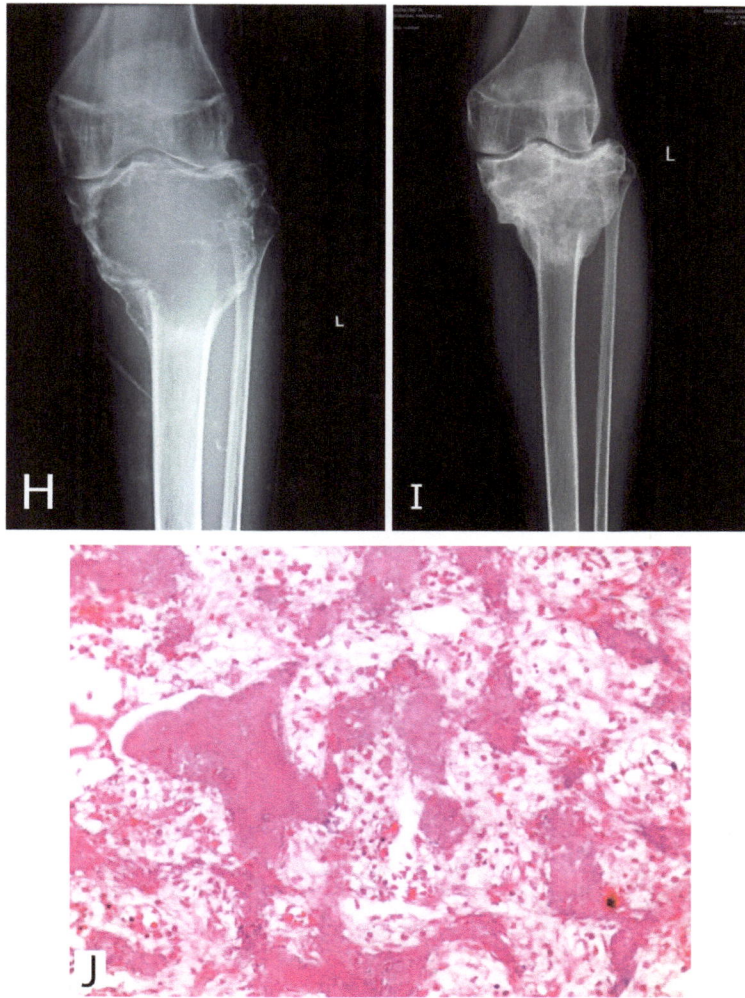

Fig. 7.5 (G) in this picture osteoid trabeculae and fibrous tissue are seen (H) abundant new bone formation with complete absence of GCT tissue following denosumab treatment (I) x-ray of left upper tibia bearing expansile destructive GCT, (J) post denosumab loss of tumor and replacement by osteoid has occurred.

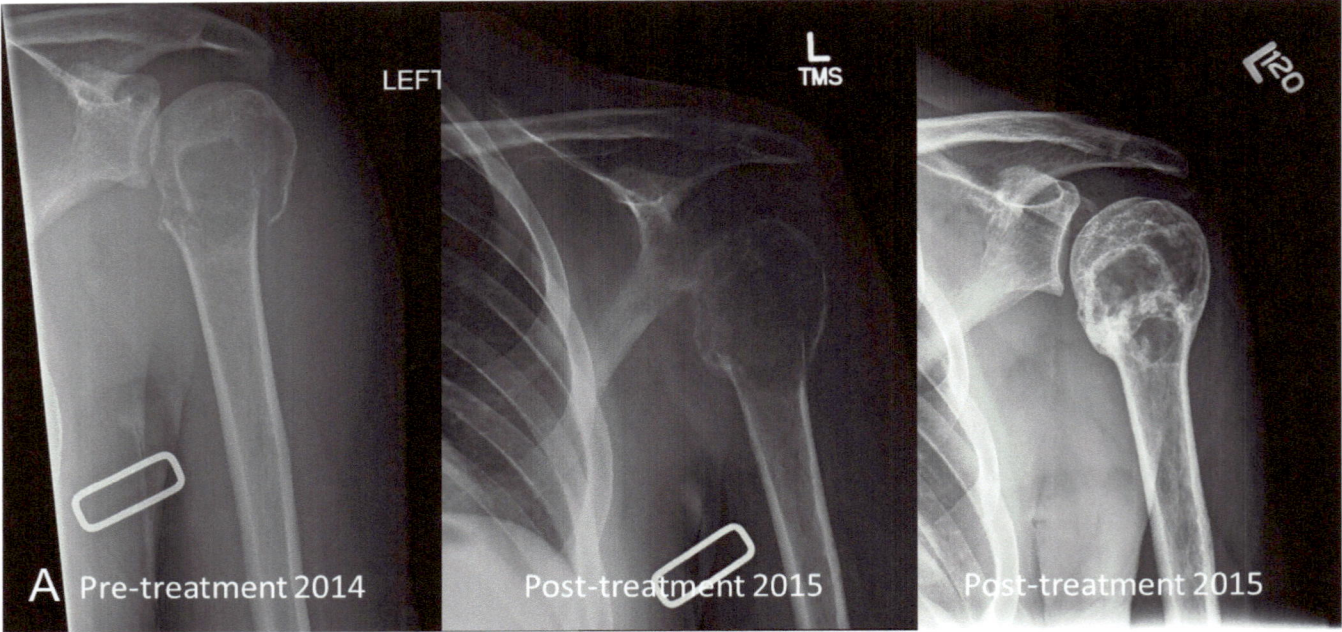

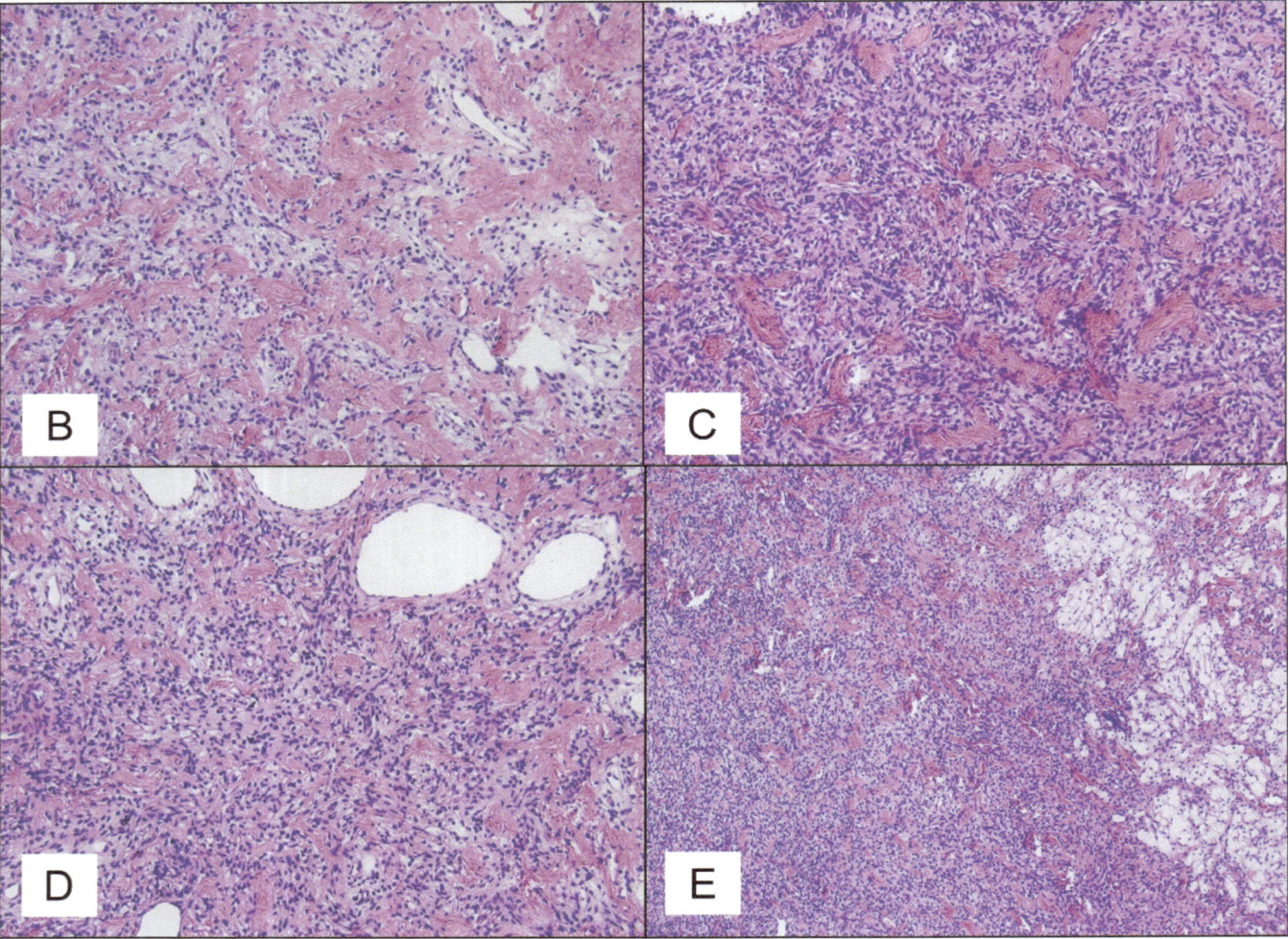

Fig. 7.6. (A) Another example of large destructive GCT involving upper end of left humerus with Denosumab treatment: Pre and post denosumab x-rays showing almost complete shrinking of the tumor and regular bone formation over 2 years of treatment (B,C,D) denosumab treatment lead to complete disappearance of osteoclasts with replacement by actively proliferating mesenchymal stromal cells, fibroblastic tissue, osteoid and foamy histiocytes (E)

References for Chapter 7

1) Fain JS, Unni KK, Beabout JW, et al. Non epiphyseal Giant cell Tumor of the Long Bones: Clinical, Radiological, and Pathologic Study. Cancer 1993; 71:3514-3519

2) Balke M, Henrichs MB, Gosheger G, et al. Giant Cell Tumors of the Axial Skeleton. Sarcoma 2012; Article ID 410973

3) Biscaglia R, Bacchini P, Pertoni F. Giant Cell Tumors of the Hand and Foot. Cancer 2000; 88:2022-2032

4) Miller J, Blank A, Yin SM, et al. A case of recurrent giant cell tumor of bone with malignant transformation and benign pulmonary metastases. Diagnostic Pathology 2010; 5:62-69

5) Dominicus M, Rugieria P, Bertoni F, et al. Histologically verified lung metastases in benign giant cell tumors-14 cases from a single institution. Int Orthop 2006; 30:499—504

6) Vishwanathan S, Jambhekar N. Metastatic Giant Cell Tumor of Bone: Are There Associated Factors and Best Treatment Modalities?

7) Caballes RL. The mechanism of metastasis in the –so-called "benign giant cell tumor of bone. Hum Pathol 1981; 12:762-767

8) Nascimento AG, Huvos AG, Marcove RC. Primary malignant giant cell tumor of bone: A Study of Eight Cases and Review of literature.

9) Bertoni F, Bacchini P, Staals EL. Malignancy in Giant Cell Tumor of Bone. Cancer 2003; 97:2520-2529

10) Wulling M, Delling G, Kaiser E. The origin of neoplastic stromal cell in giant cell tumor of bone Hum Pathol 2003; 34:983-993

11) Cowan RW, Singh G. Giant cell tumor of bone: a basic science perspective Bone 2013; 52:238-246

12) Chakarun CJ, Forrester DM, Gottsegen CJ, et al Giant cell tumor of bone: review, mimics, and new developments in treatment. Radiographics 2013; 33:197-211

13) Wojcik J, Rosenberg AE, Bredella MA, et al. Denosumab-treated giant cell tumor of bone exhibits morphologic overlap with malignant giant cell tumor of bone Am J Surg Pathol 2016; 40:72-80

Chapter 8: Chordoma

Definition

Chordoma has been described as a rare malignant tumor derived from the primitive notochord and involving the axial skeleton. It is characterized by a long clinical course, resistance to radiotherapy, and tendency to remain localized with infrequent metastasis [1].

Clinical findings

Chordoma accounts for about 5% of all primary bone tumors, usually occurs in adults with only 5% chordomas developing in patients under 20 years of age. Males are affected twice as often as females with male: female ratio of 1.8:1. According to Higginbotham et al (1967) the distribution of chordomas in the axial skeletal is 50% sacro-coccygeal, 35% sphenoid-occipital, 10% cervical and 5% thoraco-lumber with rare examples of extra notochord origin such as in the facial bones[1]. In a series of 325 cases recorded over 70-year period at the Mayo clinics, the sites of involvement were as follows: sacro-coccygeal 48.5%, sphenoid-occipital-nasal 38.5%, mobile spine 13.5% [2].

The symptoms are related to the location of the tumor. Sacral tumors give rise to constipation, urinary symptoms and, commonly pain. Ocular disturbances, cranial nerve palsy and nasal discharge typically occur in sphenoid-occipital-nasal tumors. Main symptoms in cases of vertebral tumors are pain, limitations of arms movements and loss of muscle power.

Radiological features

Osteolytic bone destruction with an adjacent soft tissue mass is the most common finding (Fig.8.1 A). There is no evidence of reactive new bone formation. Patchy calcification within the tumor parenchyma has been a frequent manifestation. MRI and CT scan have complementary role in tumor evaluation. CT evaluation is needed to assess the degree of bone involvement or destruction and to detect patterns of calcifications within the lesion. MRI provides excellent 3-dimensional analysis of the posterior fossa (especially the brainstem), cavernous sinuses, middle cranial fossa and sella turcica.

Gross

Several surgical reports are available in the literature; all show tumor extension in the surrounding tissues. The excised specimen demonstrates an encephaloid, vascular mass ranging in size from 5 cm to 20 cm) (Fig. 8.1 B, C).

Microscopic

Dahlin in his seminal work on chordomas [3] described salient histological features for diagnosis of this tumor: 1) lobular arrangement, 2) extracellular and intracellular mucus, 3) the presence of large physaliphorous cells (Fig. 8.1 D, E, F, G, 8.2 A, B, C, D, E). The latter show copious cytoplasm containing mucous droplets and is the most common and distinctive feature. The tumor cells are arranged in cords, sheets and isolated floating cells within an abundant myxoid stroma. The cuboidal epithelial-like cells display acidophilic cytoplasm and mildly atypical small nuclei. Such cells can be easily mistaken for adenocarcinoma cells. These are the typical features of a conventional chordoma and there are two variants including chondroid chordoma and dedifferentiated chordoma described below.

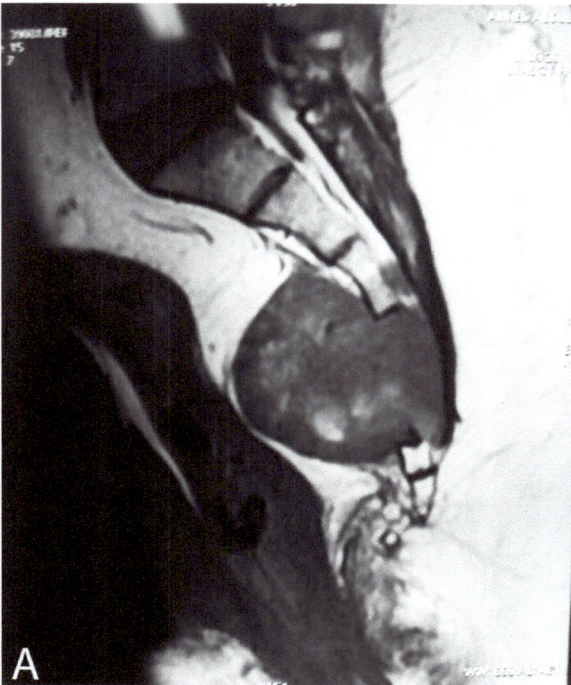

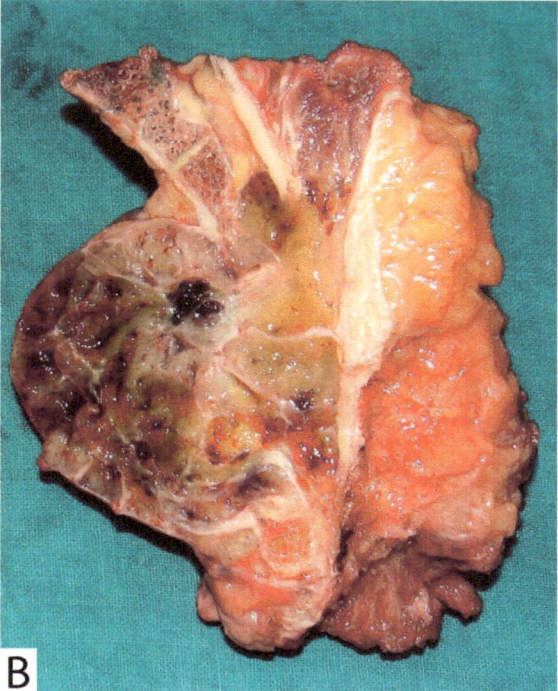

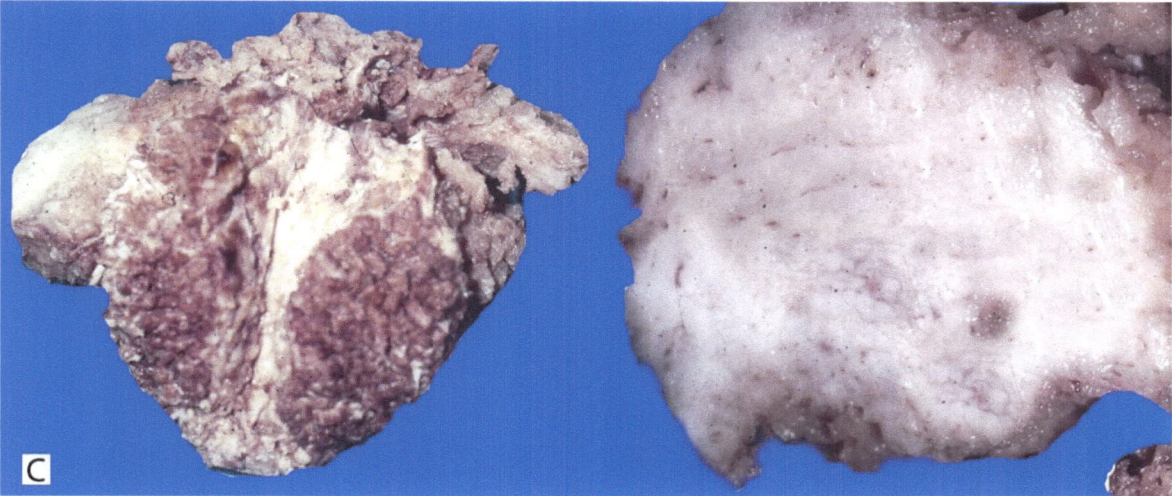

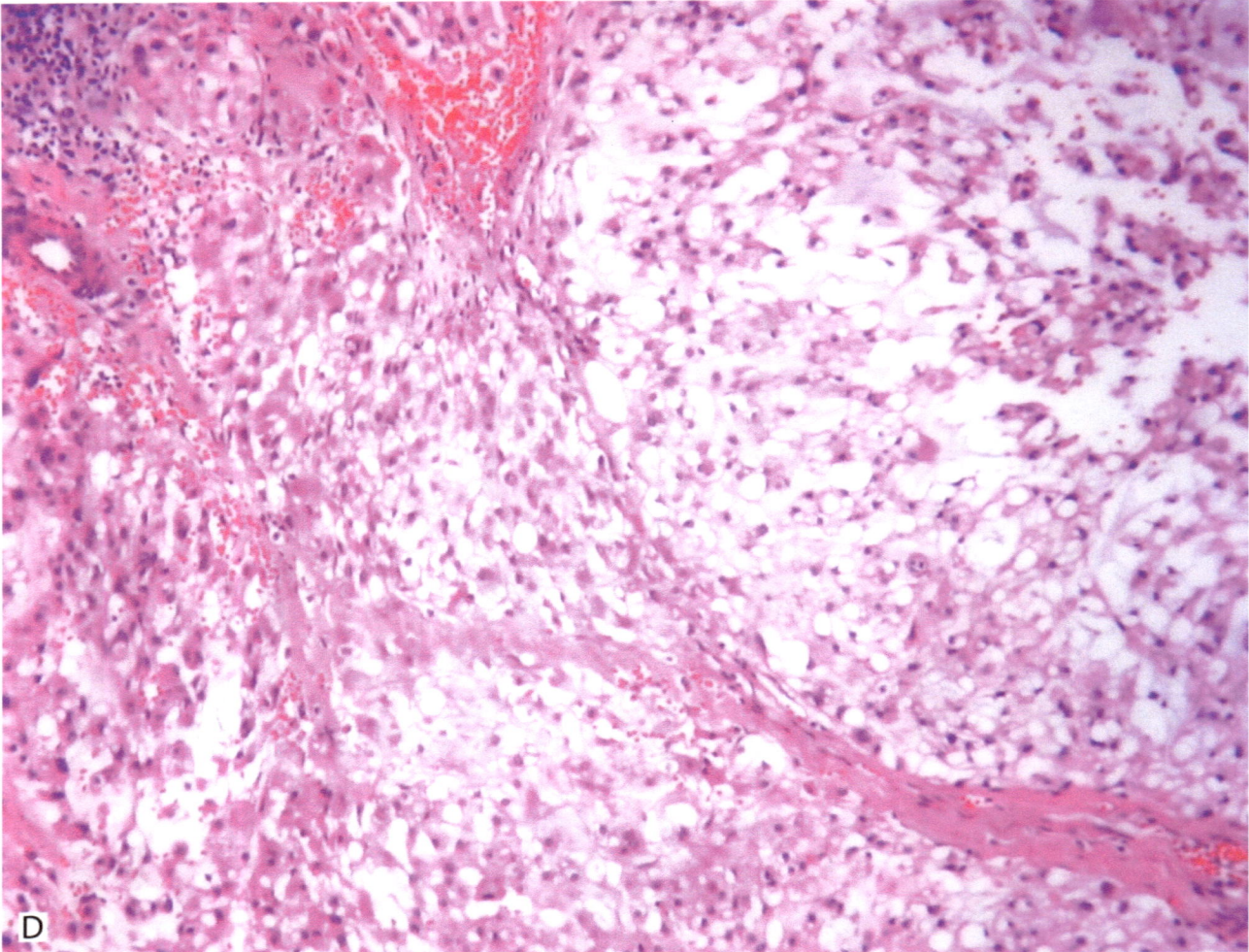

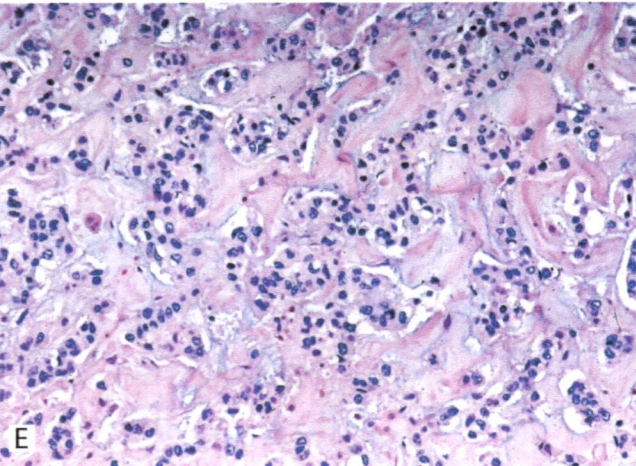

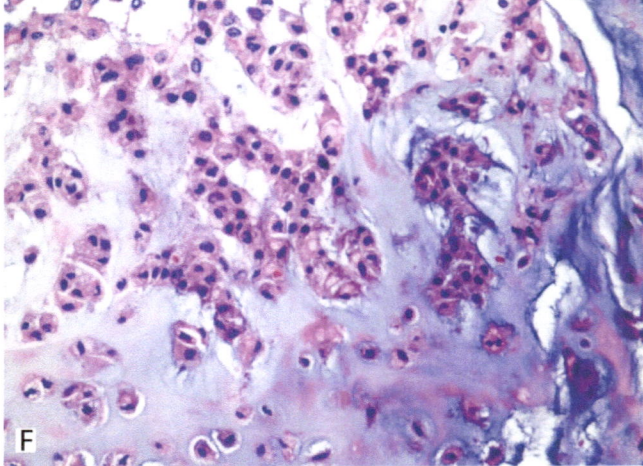

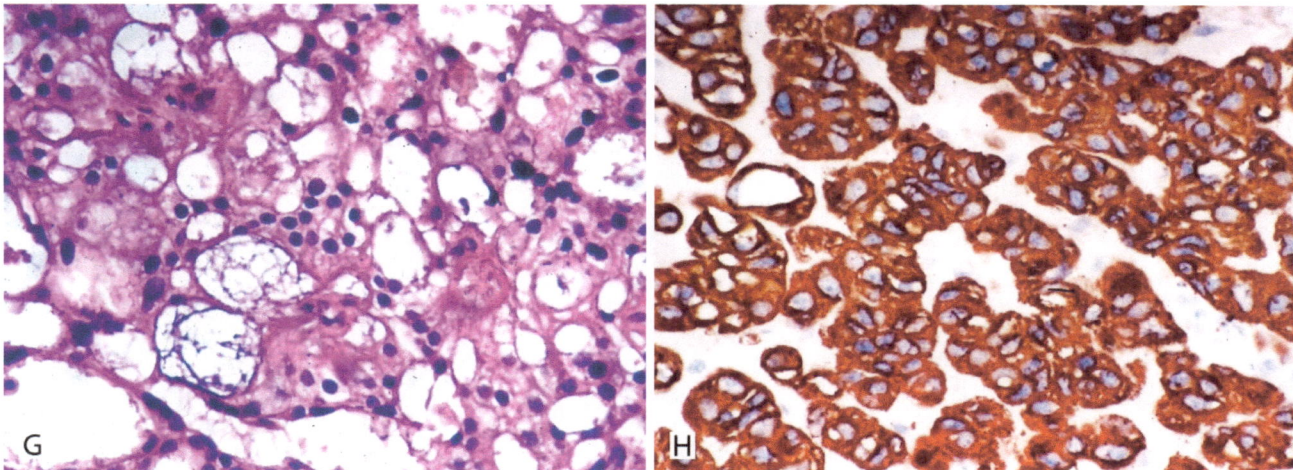

Fig. 8.1 Chordoma: a large circumscribed mass involving sacral region ;(B) excised sacrum with tumor; (C) Sacral tumor extending in to the pelvis; (D) low power view of lobulated myxoid tumor; (E , F) : cords of epithelioid tumor cells with myxoid stromal background; (G) physaliphorous cells, a hall mark of chordoma; (H) tumor cells strongly express EMA.

The differential diagnosis for chordomas involving the spine and sacrum includes metastatic adenocarcinoma. Chordomas are reactive with antibodies against S-100 protein, pan-keratin, low molecular keratin and epithelial membrane antigen (EMA) (Fig. 46 H). However, there are many tumors to be considered in the differential diagnosis, namely; extra skeletal myxoid chondrosarcoma, skeletal chondrosarcoma, dedifferentiated chondrosarcoma, mucinous adenocarcinoma etc. Only epithelial markers may not be always reliable and the problem is compounded by the small size of the available biopsy tissue.

Brachyury, a nuclear transcription factor, is a recently described immunohistochemical marker for diagnosing chordomas. Brachyury is highly expressed in all cells in nearly every chordoma. The Brachyury gene is amplified in some sporadic chordomas. Exclusive brachyury expression in more than 90% of chordomas indicates its value as a unique, specific marker in substantiating diagnosis of chordoma [4].

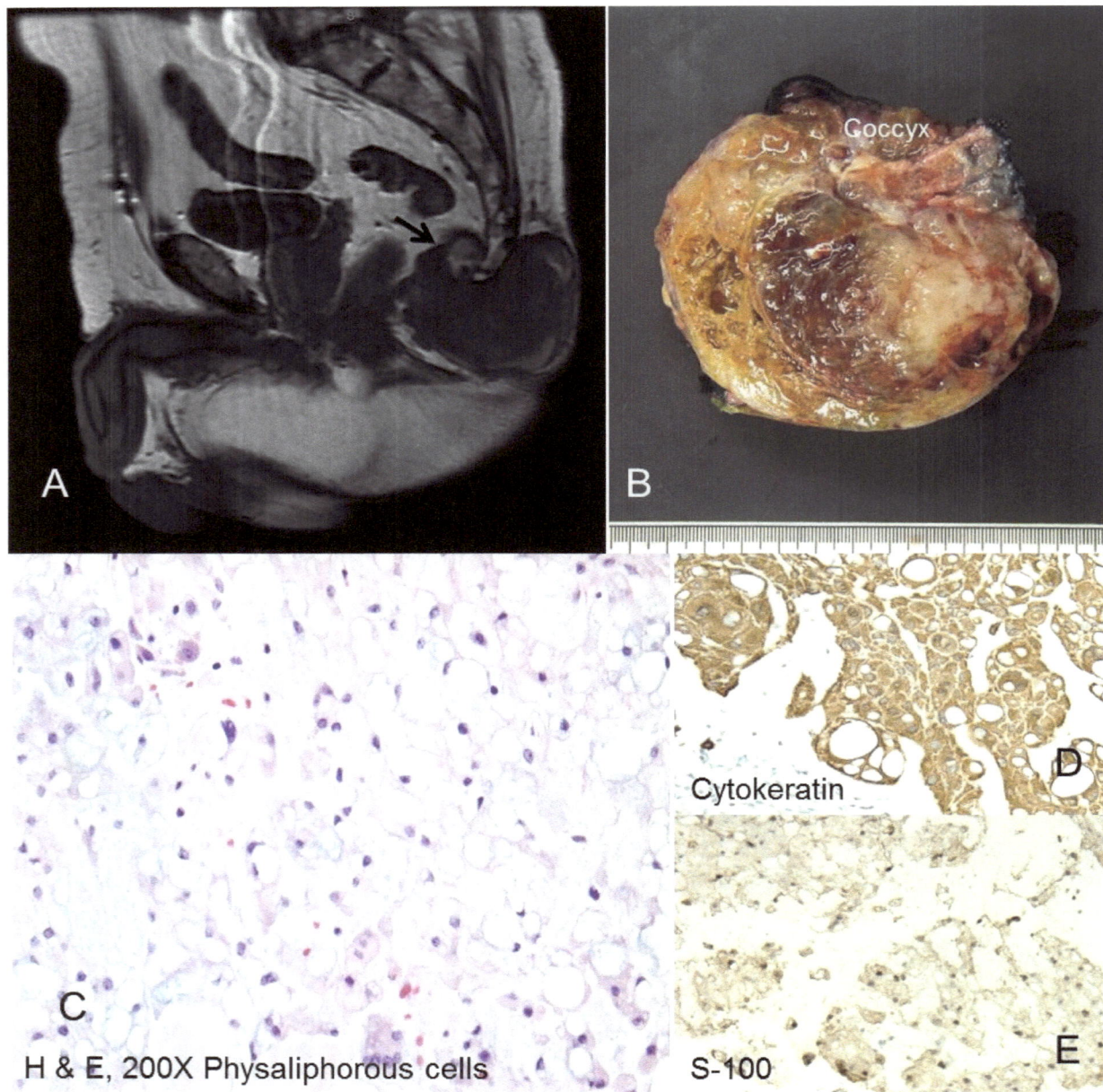

Fig. 8.2 Chordoma: a large circumscribed mass involving coccyx region ;(B) excised sacrum with tumor arising from the tip of coccyx; (c) low power view of lobulated myxoid tumor; cords of epithelioid tumor cells with myxoid stromal background and many physaliphorous cells; (D,E) tumor cells strongly express cytokeratin (AE1:AE3), S-100.

Chondroid chordoma

The tumor is composed of an admixture of chondromatous and chordomatous tissue and is usually located in the sphenoid-occipital region. Chondroid chordoma shares many of the clinical and histological features of classic chordoma and chondrosarcoma and has been shown to have better prognosis than either of the two lesions.

Electron microscopy: Certain features such as dilated RER, intracytoplasmic glycogen aggregates and abundant fibril-granular matrix are common to chordoma, chondrosarcoma, and chondroid chordoma. The presence of tonofilaments, desmosome complexes as well as complexes of RER and mitochondria were seen only in chordoma and chondroid chordoma, but not in cartilaginous tumors [5].

Dedifferentiated chordoma

Chordomas are generally regarded as tumors of low malignant potential and typically present an indolent, prolonged course of local recurrences, usually leading to fatal outcome. Metastases have been reported in 26-43% of cases[6]. In few cases, a true sarcoma has been reported to occur in conjunction with a conventional chordoma. Some dedifferentiated chordomas have occurred de novo or in recurrences; others have followed radiation therapy. Apart from the epithelial immune markers, the conventional and dedifferentiated chordomas are also stained by alpha-1 anti-chymotrypsin and vimentin [6]. Undifferentiated high grade pleomorphic sarcoma (Malignant fibrous histiocytoma) and osteosarcoma have been reported within a typical chordoma and this phenomenon heralds a poor prognosis.

Prognosis

Chordoma may respond to only wide local resection with clear margins but no response to adjuvant therapy has been reported. According to the latest and most comprehensive population-based study, the median overall survival for chordoma patients in the United States is approximately 7 years, and the overall 5, 10 and 20-year survival rates are 68%, 40% and 13%, respectively[7].

References for Chapter 8

1. Higinbotham NL, Phillips RF, Farr HW, et al. Chordoma: Thirty-five-year study at memorial hospital. Cancer 1967; 20:1841-1850
2. Volpe R, Mazabraud A. A clinicopathologic review of 25 cases of chordoma (a pleomorphic and metastasizing neoplasm) Am J Surg Pathol 1983; 7:161-170
3. Dahlin. DC and MacCarty CS. Chordoma. A study of fifty-nine cases. Cancer 1952; 5:1170-1178
4. Jambhekar NA, Rekhi B, Thorat K, et al Revisiting chordoma with Brachyury, a "New Age" Marker. Analysis of a validation study on 51 cases. Arch Pathol Lab Med 2010; 134:1181-1187
5. Valderrama E, Kahn LB, Lipper, S, et al. Chondroid Chordoma: Electron microscopy study of two cases Am J Surg Pathol 1983; 7:625-632
6. Meis JM, Raymond AK, Evans H L, et al. "Dedifferentiated" Chordoma: A clinicopathologic and immunohistochemical study of three cases. Am J Surg Pathol 1987; 22:516-525
7. McMaster ML, Goldstein AM, Bromley CM, et al, "Chordoma: incidence and survival patterns in the United States, 1973-1995.", Cancer causes & control: CCC, 2001.

Chapter 9: Adamantinoma of long bones & Osteofibrous dysplasia

Definition

Adamantinoma is a low-grade neoplasm with epithelial differentiation and a striking predilection to involve the tibia.

Clinical findings

Adamantinoma is a low grade destructive tumor that characteristically occurs in long tubular bones- anterior mid shaft of tibia in almost 90% of cases. Lower end of tibia and fibula are other sites where this tumor occurs occasionally. In a few cases tibia and fibula are involved simultaneously. Rare instances of cases occurring in femur, ulna and radius have been recorded in the literature. The tibia is involved almost exclusively, 34 of 40 cases affected tibia according to Mayo clinic data. Moon and Martin[1] collected 195 cases of well documented adamantinoma from the world literature and revealed that 85% of cases were in the tibia. The tumor is seen mainly in the young, majority being in the second and third decades. Swelling and pain are characteristic presenting symptoms in most. Not uncommonly, symptoms last for several years before medical help is sought. The frequent history of preceding trauma may indeed be important in tumor formation [1] but this theory has not many takers.

Radiology

On plain X rays the tumor presents as multiple lucent areas with sclerotic borders in the cortex, secondarily involving the medullary cavity (Fig.9.1 A). There are sclerotic areas around the lucent areas. In several cases where the lesions are restricted to cortex, the radiological features are indistinguishable from those of osteofibrous dysplasia.
Grossly the lesion appears greyish white and firm to soft.

Microscopic

This is a biphasic destructive tumor of small epithelial cells arranged in tubules, islands and slit-like spaces embedded in a mesenchymal component. Proportions of epithelial and mesenchymal components vary from case to case, and area to area. The epithelial cells may be basaloid, spindle or rarely squamous (Fig.9.1 B, C) and whatever may be epithelial pattern there is no significant atypia[2]. In some cases, slit-like spaces lined by plump cells resemble vascular spaces, though these have not been proved to be endothelial cell. The genesis of the tumor is now considered to be epithelial in origin by ultrastructural and immunohistochemical methods. The epithelial cells express cytokeratin and EMA. Hazelbag et al[3] showed that keratins 8 and 18, usually present in synovial sarcoma and metastatic carcinoma, are absent in adamantinoma.

Relation between adamantinoma and osteofibrous dysplasia

Some have pointed out association of fibrous dysplasia-like areas in adamantinoma [4]. In several cases the mesenchymal component of adamantinoma is similar to that of osteofibrous dysplasia. The radiological features and the preferential involvement of the tibia also suggest some relationship between osteofibrous dysplasia and adamantinoma[5]. It is intriguing that Hazelbag et al have reported two cases originally interpreted as osteofibrous dysplasia recurring as adamantinoma. Czerniak et al [6] proposed the existence of a continuum of fibro-osseous lesions with osteofibrous dysplasia at one end of the spectrum, classic adamantinoma at the other, and differentiated adamantinoma in the middle. It was thought that some, if not all, examples of osteofibrous dysplasia began as adamantinoma and regressed, with the reparative fibro-osseous process proliferating Osteofibrous dysplasia, which has a similar anatomic location, age distribution, and radiologic appearance as differentiated adamantinoma, may, in some cases, represent the evolution of an underlying adamantinoma.

This has raised debate regarding relationship between adamantinoma and osteofibrous dysplasia. Some authors have suggested osteofibrous dysplasia is a possible precursor of adamantinoma. In a study of 30 cases to determine whether it is a precursor lesion to adamantinoma; it was concluded that there was no conclusive evidence of a precursor role for osteofibrous dysplasia[7].

Total surgical excision is the treatment of choice. In cases where complete excision has not been achieved, high recurrence rate ranging up to 80% has been reported. Hazelbag[8] reported a local recurrence rate of 32% and metastatic rate of 29%. Recurrent tumors behave more aggressively. Rarely, there may be metastasis to inguinal lymph nodes or to lungs.

Quereshi et al[9] reported in a multicenter review of 70 cases [9] published in 2000: en bloc tumor resection with wide margins and limb salvage was shown to have 10-year survival rate of 87.2%. Amputation for adamantinoma has not been shown to improve survival when compared with the limb preserving surgery. The local recurrence rate was 8.6% at 5 years and 18.6% at 10 years. Limb salvage was attempted in 91% of patients; with final limb preservation rate of 84%. The overall mortality rate of metastasis was 13%, which is comparable to historical reports of 15% to 30%. Long-term surveillance is required for survivors of this low-grade slowly progressing tumor, for the tumor can recur after several years.

.

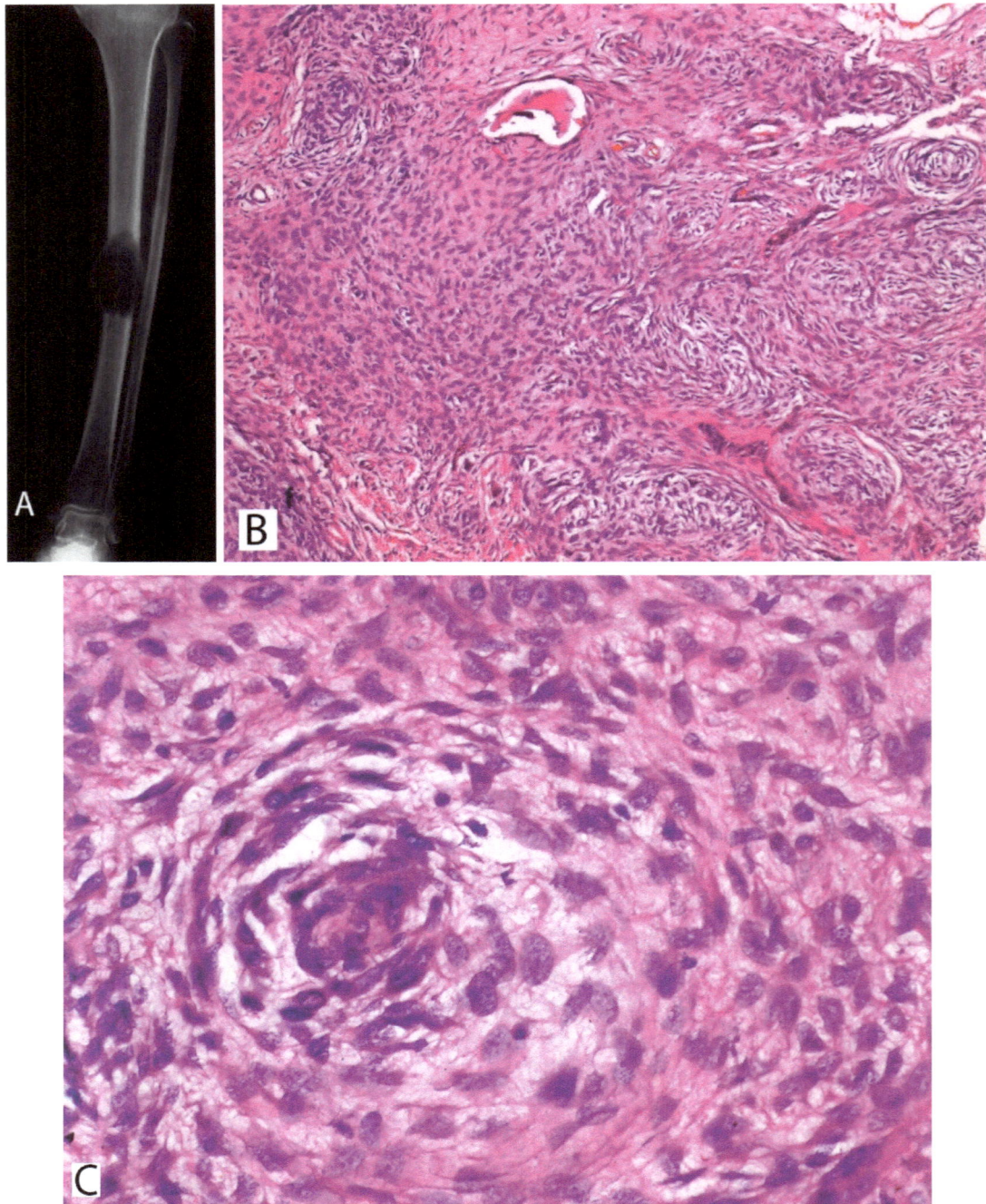

Fig. 9.1 Adamantinoma: (A) diaphyseal lytic lesion in tibia; (B, C) plump spindled cells of enamel epithelial origin in a whirling pattern, a most typical histological pattern in adamantinoma of bone. Rarely, metaplastic squamous islands may be seen.

The frequent history of preceding trauma may indeed be important in tumor formation. A high incidence of recurrence or metastases is found with inadequate cancer surgery. Known mortalities have indicated severe metastatic disease by aggressive-appearing cells. Previously, early amputation had provided good results, but wide excision or segmental resection with grafting techniques are equally successful. The recent work with allograft replacement of a widely excised segment has shown good early results.

Osteofibrous dysplasia

Definition
Osteofibrous dysplasia is a benign fibro-osseous process that exclusively involves the cortex of usually tibia, rarely fibula and occasionally both bones.

Clinical findings

Campanacci (1976) was the first to describe a distinct clinicopathologic entity, which he labeled as osteofibrous dysplasia of long bones, based on study of 39 cases (22 personal + 17 from literature). He could clearly differentiate it from the look-alike fibrous dysplasia by clinical, radiologic, histologic and clinical course. The features include age of onset either at birth or in first decade, slight male preponderance of male sex, exclusive tibial involvement, localization in mid shaft of tibial diaphysis, anterior bowing of mishit, and at times pathological fracture [10].

Although the symptoms are nonspecific, their outstanding feature is their long duration which attests to the slow rate of growth of most of these tumors. The duration of symptoms, however, was not related to prognosis[11].

Radiologically, the lesion involves mainly cortical portion, unlike fibrous dysplasia which involves medulla. The radiologic features include solitary or multiple radiolucent lesions involving the cortex of tibia (Fig.48 A). This appearance is considered to be characteristic enough to be diagnostic[11]. The lesion is usually surrounded by bony sclerosis and is situated within the expanded cortex. The "typical" roentgenogram has been previously described as a multiloculated cyst, with a soap-bubble appearance, in the mishit of the bone, or a well-defined cyst.

Histologically, it shows irregularly shaped bone trabeculae embedded within fibrous connective tissue (48 B, C). Unlike fibrous dysplasia, the trabecular bone is typically surrounded by prominent osteoblastic rimming" (Fig. 48 D, E). Campanacci and Laus described zonation with more mature bone trabeculae toward the periphery [12]. Immunoperoxidase stains show single keratin-positive cells in the majority of cases [13].

Several studies have suggested a conservative approach to management. The lesions often tend to regress with maturation of the skeleton. The current evidence indicates that surgery should not be attempted in patients less than 10 years of age [14].

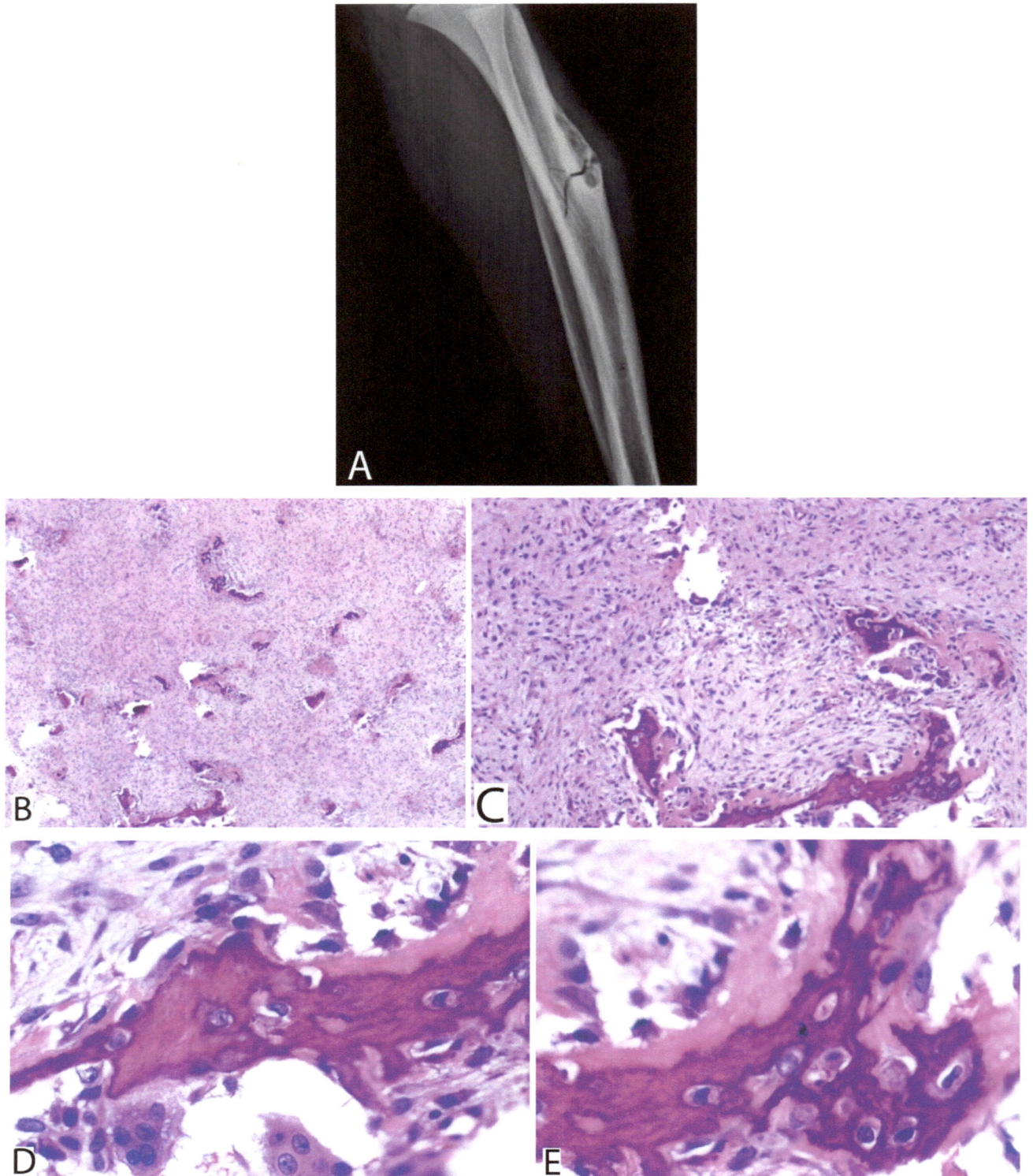

Fig.49. (A) X ray: a case of osteofibrous dysplasia note pathologic fracture at the site of cortical lucency in the upper diaphysis of tibia; (B, C) scanner and low power views show short, irregular osteoid trabeculae widely separated by broad zones of small spindly fibroblasts, note close resemblance to fibrous dysplasia; D, E) quite plump osteoblasts in osteoid trabeculae

References for Chapter 9

Adamantinoma

1) Moon NE, Mori H. Adamantinoma of the appendicular skeleton-updated. Clin Orthop 1986; 204:215-237
2) Weiss SW, Dorfman HD. Adamantinoma of long bone. Analysis of nine new cases with emphasis on metastasizing lesions and fibrous dysplasia-like changes Hum Pathol 1977; 8:141-153
3) Hazelbag HM, Fleuren GJ, vd Broek LJ et al. Adamantinoma of long bones: keratin subclass immunoreactive pattern with reference to its histogenesis. Am J Surg Pathol1993; 17:1225-1233
4) Baker PL, Dockerty MB, Coventry. Adamantinoma of long bones: review of the literature and a report of three new cases J Bone Joint Surg AM1954; 36:704-720
5) Cohen DM, Dahlin DC, Pugh DG. Fibrous dysplasia associated with adamantinoma of the long bones Cancer 1962; 15:515-521
6) Czerniak B, Rojas-Corona RR, Dorfman HD et al Morphological diversity of long bone adamantinoma. The concept of differentiated (regressing) adamantinoma and its relationship to osteofibrous dysplasia Cancer 1989; 64:2319-2334
7) Jain D, Jain VK, Vashishta RK, et al. Adamantinoma: A clinicopathologic review and update. Diagnostic Pathology 2008; 3.8
8. Hazelbag HM, Taminiau AH, Fleuren GJ, et al. Adamantinoma of long bones. A clinicopathologic study of 32 patients with emphasis on histological subtype, precursor lesion, and biological behavior J Bone Joint Surg 1994; 76:1482-1499
9. Qureshi AA, Shott S, Mallin BA, Gitelis S. Current trends in the management of adamantinoma of long bones. An international study J Bone Joint Surg Am. 2000; 82:1122–31.

Osteofibrous dysplasia

10. Campanacci M. Osteofibrous dysplasia of long bones: a new clinical entity Ital. J Orthop Tramadol 1976; 2:221-237
11. Unni K K, Dahlin DC, Beabout JW Adamantinoma of long bones Cancer 1974; 34:1796-1805
12. Campanacci M, Laus M Osteofibrous dysplasia of the tibia and fibula J Bone Joint Surg Am 1981; 63:367-375
13. Sweet DE, Vinh TN, Devaney K. Cortical osteofibrous dysplasia of long bone and its relationship to adamantinoma. A clinicopathologic study of 30 cases Am J Surg Pathol 1992; 16:282-290
14. Nakashima Y, Yamamuro T, Fujiwara Y, et al. Osteofibrous dysplasia (Ossifying fibroma of long bones): A study of 12 cases

Chapter 10: Tumor-like lesions of bone

Giant cell reparative granuloma
Aneurysmal bone cyst (ABC) and Solid ABC
Hyperparathyroidism
Paget's disease
Phosphaturic Mesenchymal tumor

Giant cell reparative granuloma (GCRG)

Giant cell reparative granulomas are benign, osteolytic, non-neoplastic, granulomatous lesions of bone, which occur most commonly in the maxilla and mandible in children and young adults. It is solitary, expanded lesion and infrequently may extend into the surrounding soft tissue [1].
Lesions occurring outside jaw bones are reported in many sites: hand and feet (10.1 A), axial skeleton, long bones, facial bones, orbit and nasal sinuses.

Jamil et al [2] reported a large mass of GCRG occupying sphenoid sinus, sella turcica and encroaching upon dorsum sella and clivus with bony erosion. The patient presented with long standing headache and diplopia. This case is an example of a locally invasive lesion, which is universally considered to be a non-neoplastic reactive lesion yet can be quite destructive locally. In this case patient responded well to a thorough local curettage.
Etiology of GCRG is not known but it is believed that trauma is the most likely cause. Other proposed etiologies include development anomalies, hormonal influences, and infection [3].

Microscopic

The features include variable number of small-sized osteoclastic type giant cells arranged in a vaguely clustered manner in a fibrogenic stroma exhibiting focal collagenization. Reactive new bone formation with cystic areas and evidence of old hemorrhage are present. In some fields, the number of osteoclastic giant cells may be quite large, creating suspicion of GCT. Fibrogenic stroma is a defining feature of giant cell reparative granuloma, easily distinguishing it from mesenchymal stroma of GCT (Fig. 10.1 B, C, D). Differential diagnosis includes true giant cell tumor, brown tumor of hyperthyroidism, ABC, cherubism etc. Lesions similar to giant cell reparative granulomas when they occur in bones other than jaw are called solid aneurysmal bone cysts.

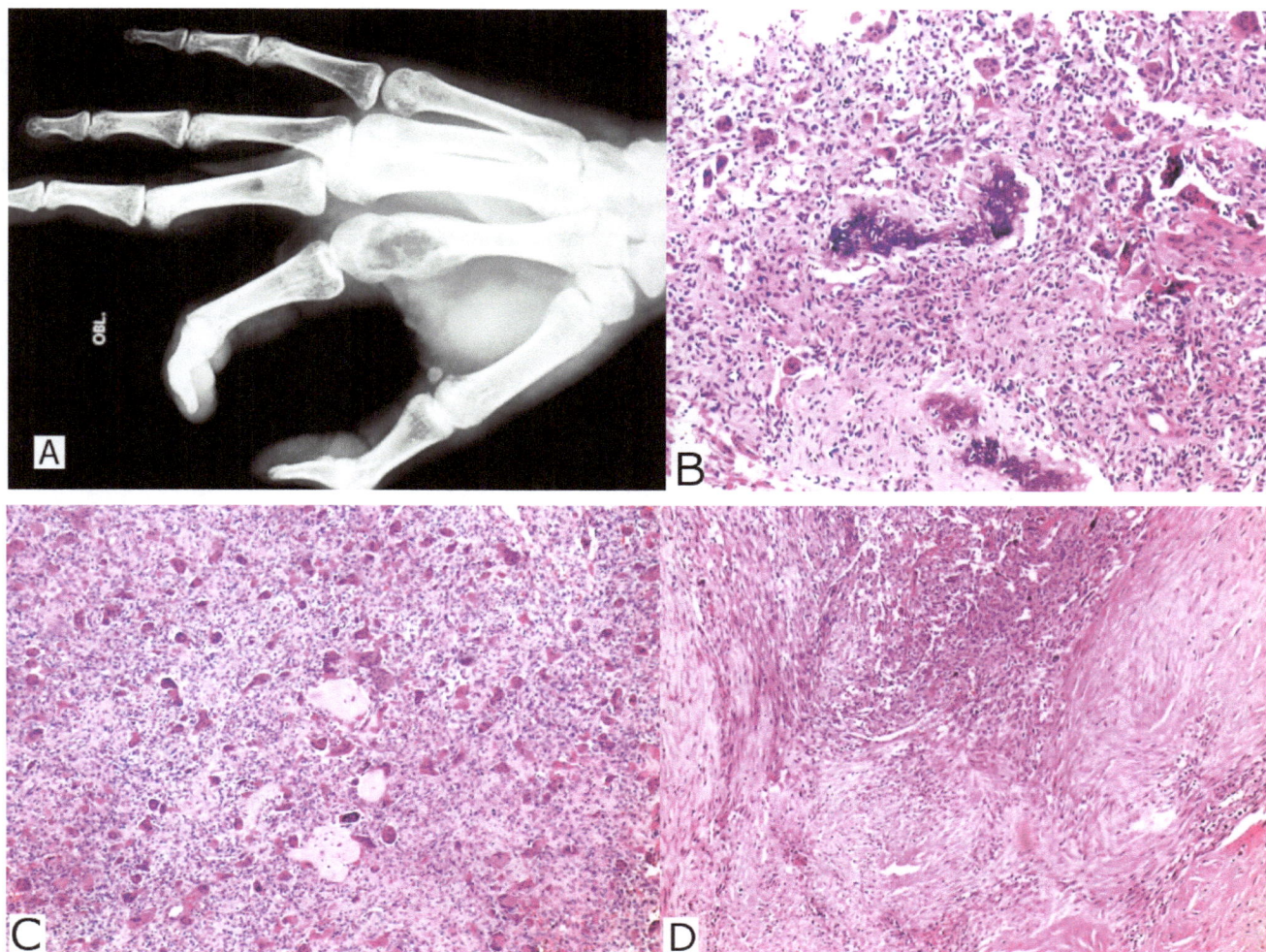

Fig. 10.1 A) Giant cell reparative granuloma: lytic lesion in the head of metacarpal bone in epiphyseal-metaphyseal region; (B) Giant cell reparative granuloma with newly formed bone and 'chondroid aura' that is usually seen in aneurysmal bone cyst; (C) abundant collagen forming spindle cells and few small giant cells; (D) abundant reactive focally hyalinized fibroblastic tissue and a patch of chronic inflammatory cells

Giant cell reparative granuloma of bones of hand and foot

In a review of 30 cases of GCRG of hand and foot, Ostrovasky et al reported that lesions of florid reactive periosteitis, bizarre parosteal osteochondromatous proliferation (Nora's lesion), and giant cell reparative granuloma made up larger percentage of these lesions in hand and foot than bone at any other site [4].

GRCG of jaw bones and extra gnathic bones

In one publication[5], 22 cases of GCRG in jaw bones were compared with 67 cases of extra gnathic bones. Females were affected twice as frequently as males in both groups and there was no variation in age of occurrence. Small bones of hand and foot (17+16 =33 cases) were the most common sites in extra gnathic bones. Histology of extra gnathic lesions was closely similar with that of lesions of jaw bone

Aneurysmal bone cyst (ABC)

Clinical findings

General consensus today is that ABC is a reactive lesion and not a neoplasm. This is a rare disease accounting for about 2 % of the bone tumors and tumor-like lesions. Almost 80% of the cases occur in those younger than 20 years of age. Though it may occur in any bone, metaphysis of long tubular bones, mainly around the knee, craniofacial bones and posterior elements of vertebrae are common sites. Small bones of hands and feet, and tarsal and calcaneal bones are affected, although much less commonly. There is no gender predilection. Symptoms mainly are of pain and swelling. Rarely pathologic fracture may be the presenting symptom. Vertebral lesions may present various neurological deficits caused by cord compression.

In 238 patients with ABC studied in the Mayo Clinic, more than 80% of the lesions were in long bones, flat bones, or the spinal column. Of the lesions initially treated at the Mayo Clinic, 95% were typical ABC; the rest were "solid" variants. Except for the absence of obvious cavernous channels and spaces, there was no significant histologic difference between solid variant and typical ABC[6].

X-rays (Fig 10.2 A, B, C, G) characteristically show blow out expansion of bone situated eccentrically in the medullary cavity. Rarely the lesion may be situated even in the cortex or periosteum. The lesion tends to grow rapidly; the cortex may be destroyed, and the lesion may bulge out into the soft tissue. CT is quite helpful; it highlights the peripheral bone shell and demonstrates fluid-fluid levels in the lesion [7].

Gross

When the lesions are totally excised, dilated vascular spaces filled with blood are seen replacing the bone. The lesions are more often curetted and the curetted material appears soft, membranous, and reddish brown (Fig 10.2 D, E).

Microscopic

Essentially the lesion is composed of several large cystic "vascular" spaces filled with blood. The septa separating the spaces show loosely arranged fibroblasts, capillaries, scattered or clustered multinucleated giant cells, hemosiderin pigment deposits and reactive new bone. All these features essentially suggest a reactive process (Fig 10.2 F, H). The spindled fibroblasts in the cyst wall appear to be the basic pathologic component, which may show regular mitotic activity. This spindle cell component may be similar to that in nodular fasciitis. At times, there may be osteoclastic giant cells in large compact sheets, almost indistinguishable from giant cell tumor.

In most aneurysmal bone cysts there is solid portions showing fibroblastic proliferation with reactive new bone and scattered multinucleated giant cells. In several cases there are bands of stromal mineralization giving the structure chondroid aura[6], considered to be characteristic feature of aneurysmal bone cyst.

ABC has been difficult to differentiate from telangiectatic osteosarcoma. Every case of ABC should be studied carefully to rule out telangiectatic osteosarcoma. Both occur commonly in the metaphysis of long bones, affect the same age group and radiologically are indistinguishable from each other. Even histologically there is overlap between the two. Areas like ABC are common in telangiectatic osteosarcoma. The only difference between the two is presence of atypical cells at least focally in the septa. Unless looked for carefully, these atypical cells may be missed altogether. Rarely atypical cells may be seen only in blood clots within the cyst.

Secondary aneurysmal bone cyst

About 50% of aneurysmal bone cysts occur secondary to some underlying pathology, mainly neoplastic [8]. Martinez and Sissons [9] reported that 28% of 123 ABCs were secondary.

Giant cell tumor
Chondroblastoma
Osteoblastoma
Chondromyxoid fibroma
Fibrous dysplasia
Giant cell tumors commonly show aneurysmal bone cyst-like changes. Moreover, in few cases of ABC, areas indistinguishable from GCT are seen. Hence histological differentiation between these two lesions becomes important, and may be difficult. The clues to differentiate one from the other, include age and site (metaphyseal or epiphyseal).

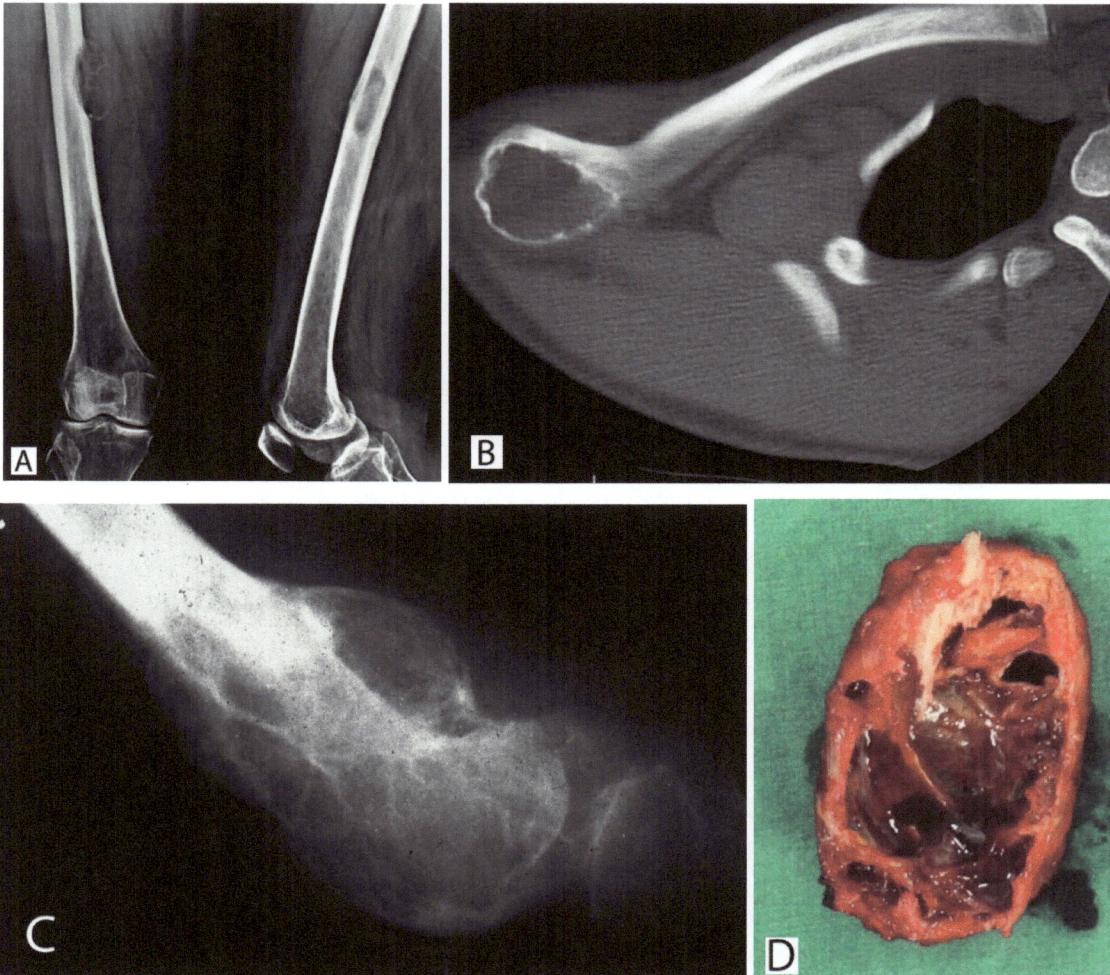

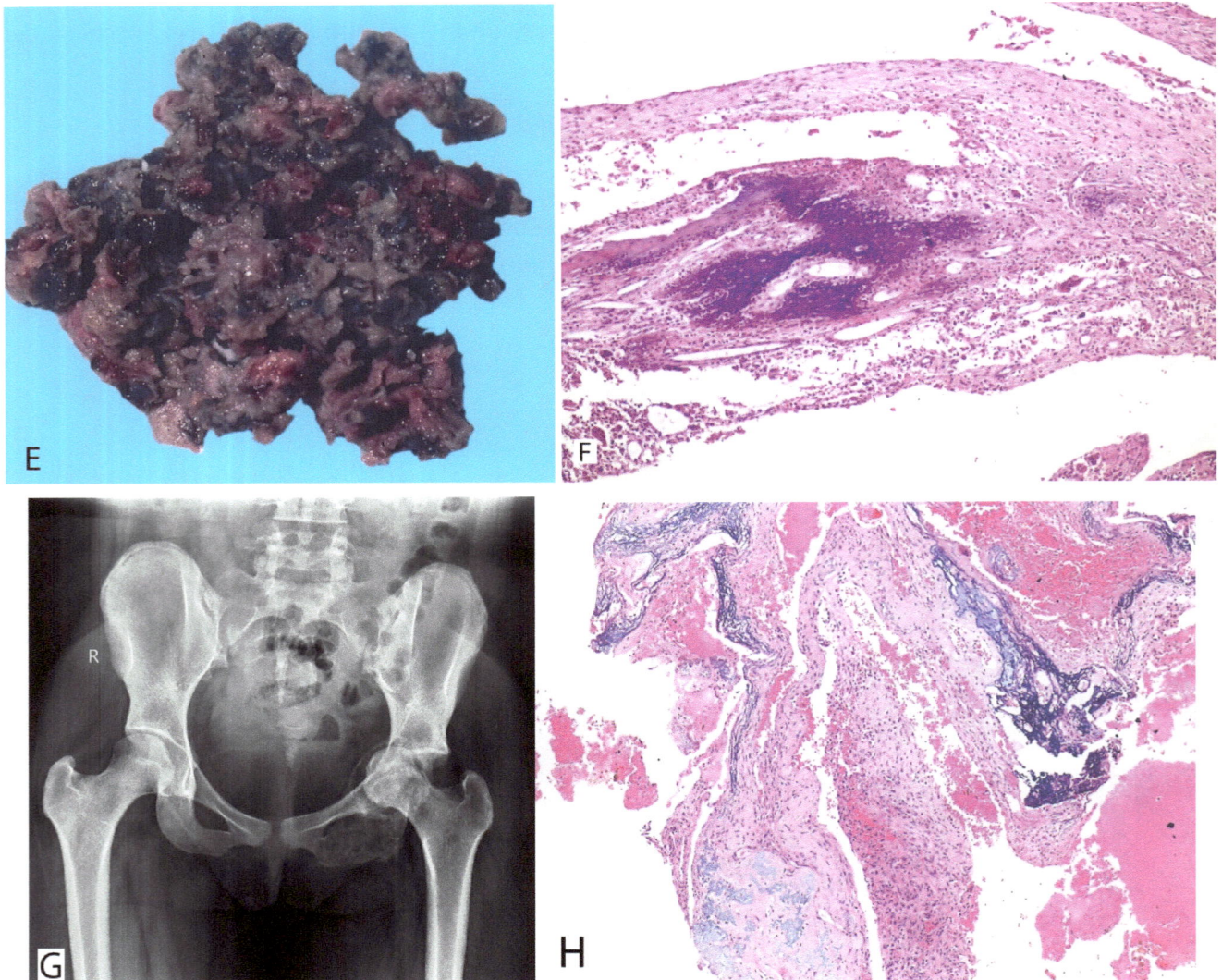

Fig. 10.2 (A) Aneurysmal bone cyst: subperiosteal lytic expansile lesion in the diaphysis of femur; (B) Aneurysmal bone cyst: lateral end of right clavicle (C) cystic blow out lesion involving metaphysio-epiphyseal region of humerus ;D) circumscribed mass from case C: large blood filled cysts separated by thick partly osseous septa; (E) curetted material from a large cystic lesion in upper metaphysis of femur, note open ends of multiple cysts appearing like large blood vessels; (F) elongated dilated blood containing cysts separated by very thick fibrous septa containing few small osteoclasts and dark blue mineralized areas with chondroid aura; (G) ischium enlarged with a radiolucent mass; (H) Aneurysmal bone cyst with bands of calcium and chondroid tissue in septa enclosing blood filled cysts

Solid Aneurysmal Bone Cyst

Though cystic spaces filled with blood constitute striking feature of aneurysmal bone cysts, cysts do not represent a component of the basic pathology. Not uncommonly these lesions are composed mainly of solid portions without cystic areas, and are recognized as 'solid' aneurysmal bone cysts. The lesions are morphologically similar to giant cell reparative granulomas. Sanerkin et al [10] reported in 1983, four examples of an unusual non-cystic intraosseous lesion which did not confirm to hitherto recognized entity and, which can be mistaken for a variety of other conditions including sarcoma and giant cell tumor. It was histologically characterized by florid fibroblastic and fibrohistiocytic proliferation, focal aggregates of osteoclasts, osteoblastic differentiation with osteoid production and occasional foci of degenerate calcifying fibromyxoid tissue with a "chondroid aura". This constellation of histological features is seen in patches in the conventional ABC. The authors called this lesion 'solid aneurysmal bone cyst", a term almost universally accepted now. Bertoni et al alternatively call solid aneurysmal bone cyst (ABC), as giant cell reparative granuloma of long bones [11]. Of the 200 cases of ABC studied in this series only 15 cases were both grossly and microscopically solid variants

Though reactive in nature, this is locally destructive. Total surgical extirpation is the treatment of choice; when this is not feasible because of anatomical constraints, curetting is done. Several of these tend to recur. Savardekar and others reported a case of solid ABC as giant cervical spinal mass and commented on spinal Solid ABC cases. The spine is very rarely affected, with only 15 cases reported in the literature. Solid ABCs have been known to occur exclusively in the pediatric age group, with a predilection for the female sex. Half of the reported cases have occurred in the thoracic spine [12].

Hyperparathyroidism / Brown tumor:

Hyperparathyroidism may present as a primary bone tumor, both radiologically (Fig 10.3 A, B) and histologically. Majority of cases present as cystic lesion with fibro-osseous and giant cell components ("osteitis fibrosa cystic"). Hypercalcemia and elevation of serum parathormone are the best indicator of the disease. A high index of suspicion is required for a clinical diagnosis of hyperparathyroidism.

Subperiosteal resorption along the lateral aspects of the middle phalanges of the index, middle and ring fingers are findings virtually pathognomic of hyperparathyroidism[13]. Subperiosteal resorption may be evident in symphysis pubis, clavicles, ischial tuberosity, scapula and vertebrae. Loss of lamina dura surrounding the tooth roots has been described in many cases [13].

Any fibro-osseous lesion in the bone with atypical features, which cannot be neatly categories into one or other known entities, hyperparathyroidism should be suspected. The brown tumor (Fig 10.3 C) of hyperparathyroidism may closely resemble the solid variant of aneurysmal bone cyst [14]; hence before making this diagnosis it is mandatory to carry out tests of serum calcium and parathormone levels. Histologically, extensive bone loss with replacement by cellular fibroblastic tissue, numerous osteoclastic giant cells and pockets of hemosiderin deposits are seen. Bone regeneration in the form of lamellar bone trabeculae covered with a broad layer of unmineralized osteoid is often seen. (Fig 10.3 D, E).

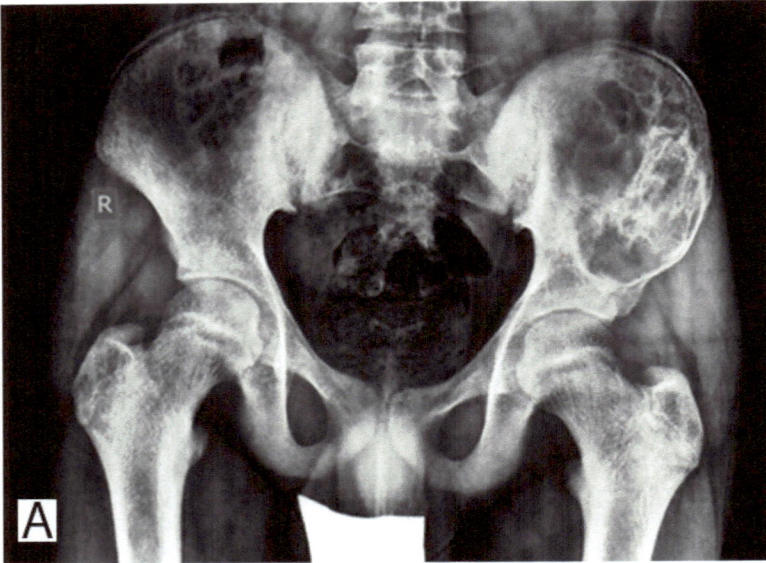

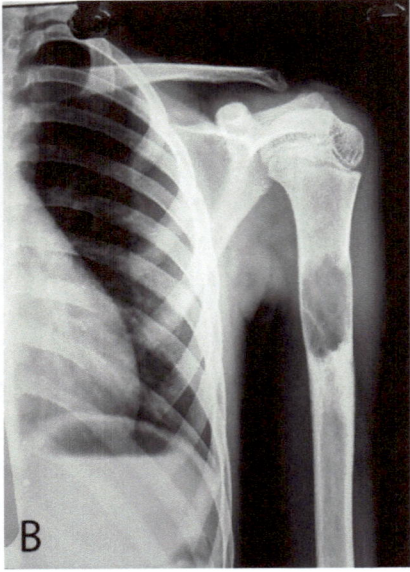

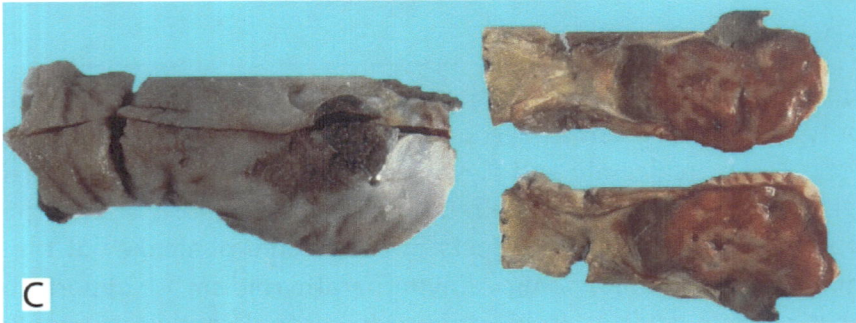

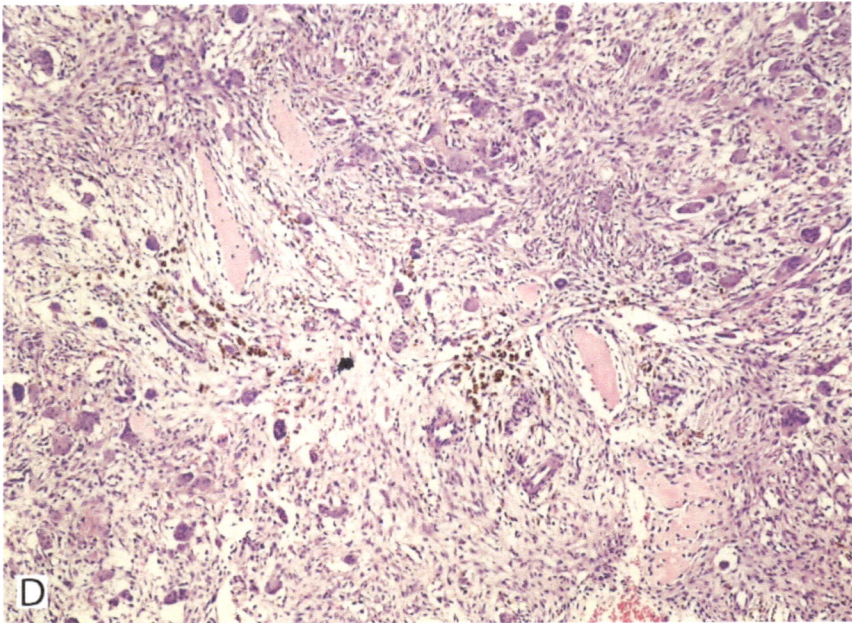

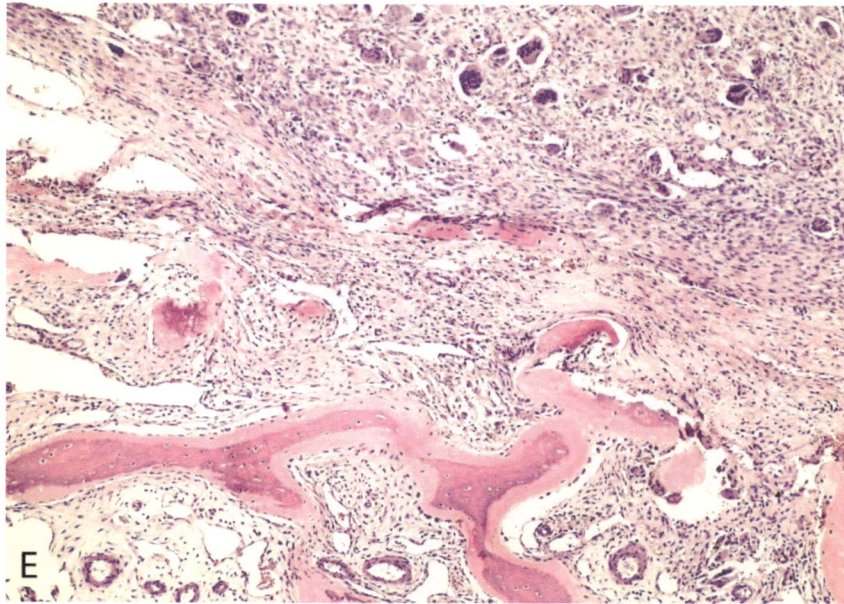

Fig. 10.3 1Hyperparathyroidism: (A&B) multiple "cystic" lesions in pelvis & humerus; (C) one patient presented with nonhealing deep ulcer requiring amputation, bones show "brown tumor" (D) extensive bone loss with replacement by cellular fibroblastic tissue, numerous osteoclastic giant cells and pockets of hemosiderin deposits; (E) in this illustration, apart from findings seen in earlier picture, bone regeneration in the form of lamellar bone trabeculae covered with a broad layer of unmineralized osteoid is evident

Paget's disease of bone:

Clinical findings

Paget's disease of bone is a peculiar structural abnormality of osteolytic and osteoblastic remodeling of bone trabeculae. It occurs in older patients, 90% of patients with Paget's disease are over 55 years of age. It has a very unusual geographic distribution, and highest incidence has been reported in England, Australia and Western Europe[15]. While in India this disease is extremely rare, although not unheard of. The most common sites are lumbosacral spine, pelvis and skull, and less commonly long bones of limbs and jaw bones. The disease is usually polyostotic with marked elevations of serum alkaline phosphatase levels. The latter may be normal in mono-ostotic disease. Patients complain of thickening of bones but are otherwise asymptomatic for years. Later, the patients present with increasing bone pain, skeletal deformities and fractures.

Radiology

The x-ray appearance of Paget's disease corresponds to the phase of the disease and therefore includes a spectrum of lytic, mixed lytic and sclerotic, and diffusely sclerotic findings; the disease always extends to the end of the bone. Both, cortical and medullary bones are thickened and irregular. The demarcation between normal bone and afflicted bone is quite sharp and pointed. Early changes in skull bones reveal well defined radiolucent defects and later changes include thickening of bones with increased radiodensity and "cotton wool" appearance[16]. Fractures of the long tubular bones are characteristically transverse and are associated with excessive callus formation (Fig.10.4 A, B, C, D, E).

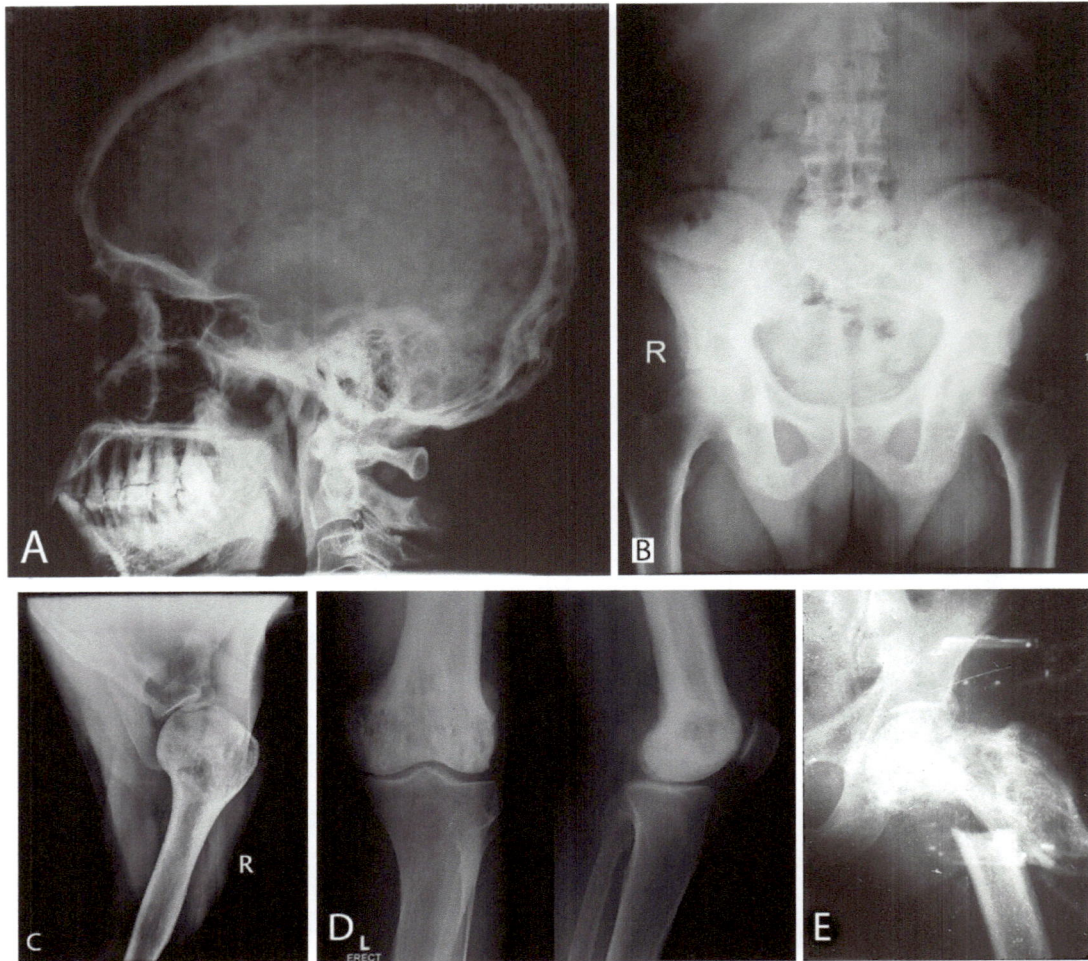

Fig.10.4 Paget's disease: (A&B) densely sclerotic skull bones and pelvis with" cotton wool" appearance; (C&D) sclerotic limb bones, particularly femur; (E) thick sclerotic bone with fracture; bones may be quite thick but fracture can and do occur easily

Microscopic

The osteolytic phase reveals highly vascular fibrous connective tissue filling the marrow cavity. This is accompanied by active osteoclastic resorption and prominent new bone formation. In the osteoblastic phase uneven trabecular widening occurs. Accentuation of cement lines with mosaic pattern represents a diagnostic feature (Fig. 10.5 A, B, C).

Secondary osteosarcoma occurs in Paget's disease after a long latent period of 8 to 16 years. Fibrosarcoma, undifferentiated pleomorphic sarcoma, and giant cell tumor (Fig.10.6) are also reported. A case of malignant lymphoma has also been recorded in the background of Paget's disease.

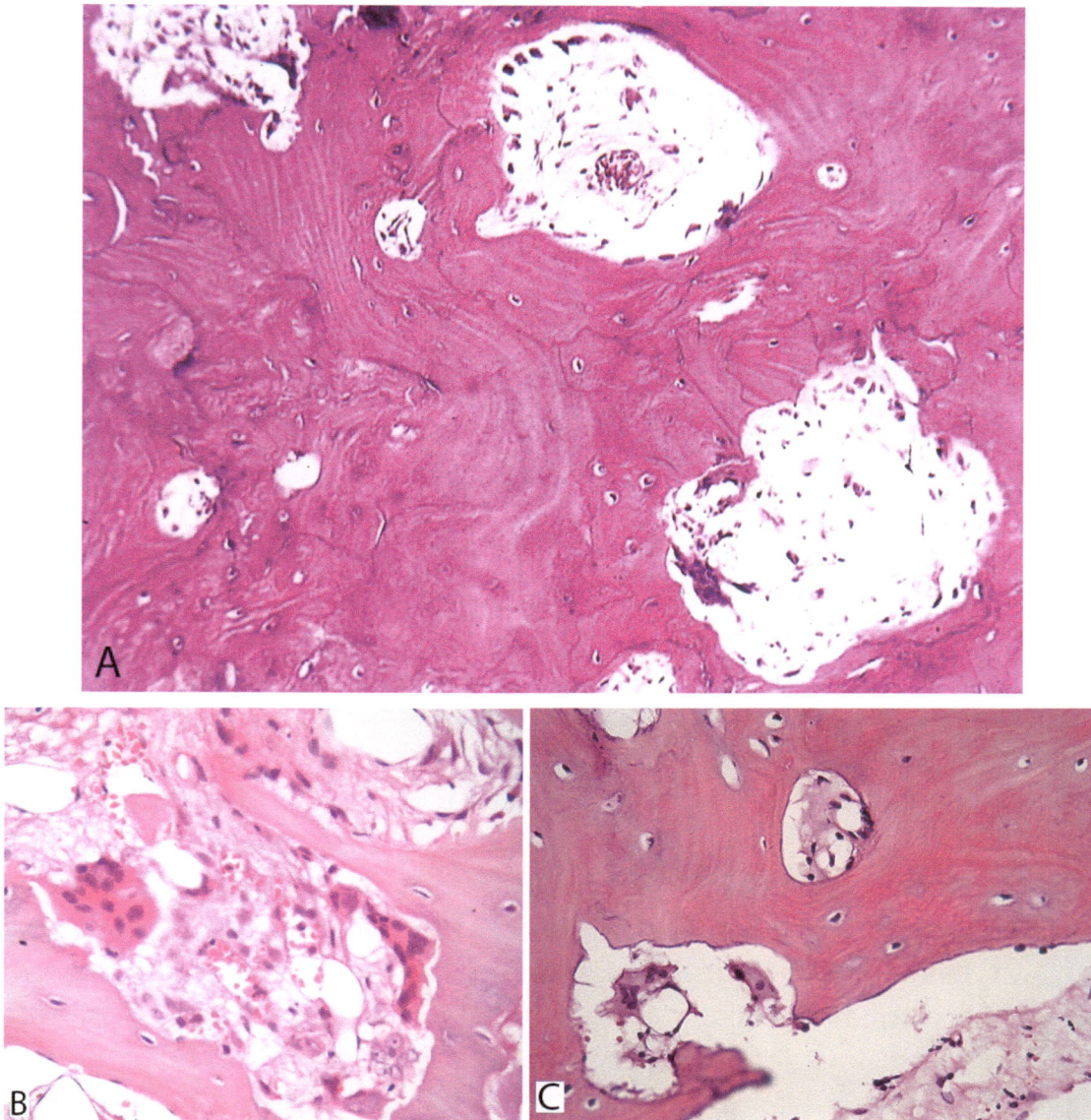

Fig. 10.5 Paget's disease of bones: (A) osteoblastic phase with very irregular widening of mosaic trabecular plate showing many cement lines (regeneration and repair); (B) bone trabeculae show ragged borders due to osteoclastic resorption; (C) thickened bone with a single deep Howship's cavernous lacuna containing two osteoclastic cells, this is the basic lesion of Paget's disease.

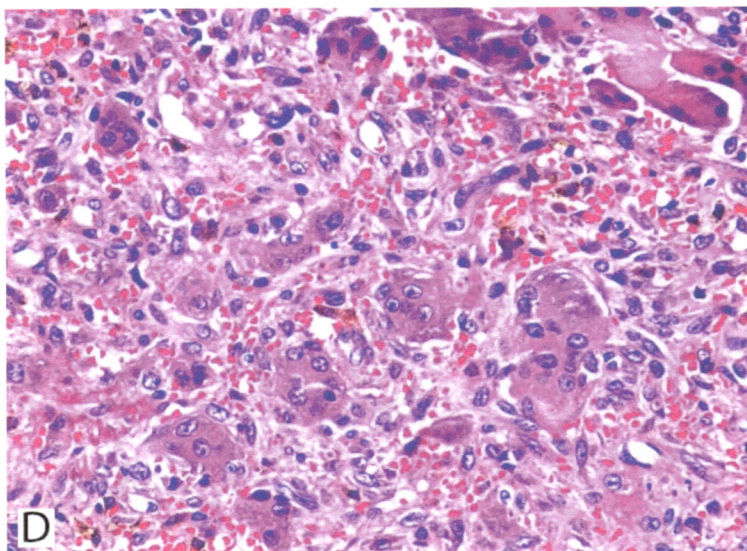

Fig. 10.6 Giant cell tumor associated with Paget's disease

Phosphaturic mesenchymal tumor of bone

A very rare mesenchymal tumor, occurring in both soft tissue and bone, may be associated with osteomalacia, has been known for more than five decades. The term phosphaturic mesenchymal tumor–mixed connective tissue type (PMT-MCT) has been proposed for these tumors. In 2004 Folpe et al [17] reported 32 cases (29 associated with oncogenic osteomalacia, and three without osteomalacia, but with characteristic histology), and reviewed 109 cases previously reported in the literature. They confirmed the view proposed earlier that oncogenic–osteomalacia associated mesenchymal tumors are a single histological entity, and are characterizes by 'low cellularity, myxoid change, bland spindle cells, distinctive "grungy" calcified matrix, fat, microcysts, hemorrhage, osteoclasts, and an incomplete membrane ossification'. A small number of these oncogenic-osteomalacia associated tumors do not show these characteristic features, but may be classified as other already known histological entities, both of soft tissue and bone.

While majority of these occur in soft tissue, a small number involves bone. While most are benign tumors histologically and biologically, a few are cellular and atypical (10.7 A, B, C) and a rare one behaves aggressively and even metastasize.

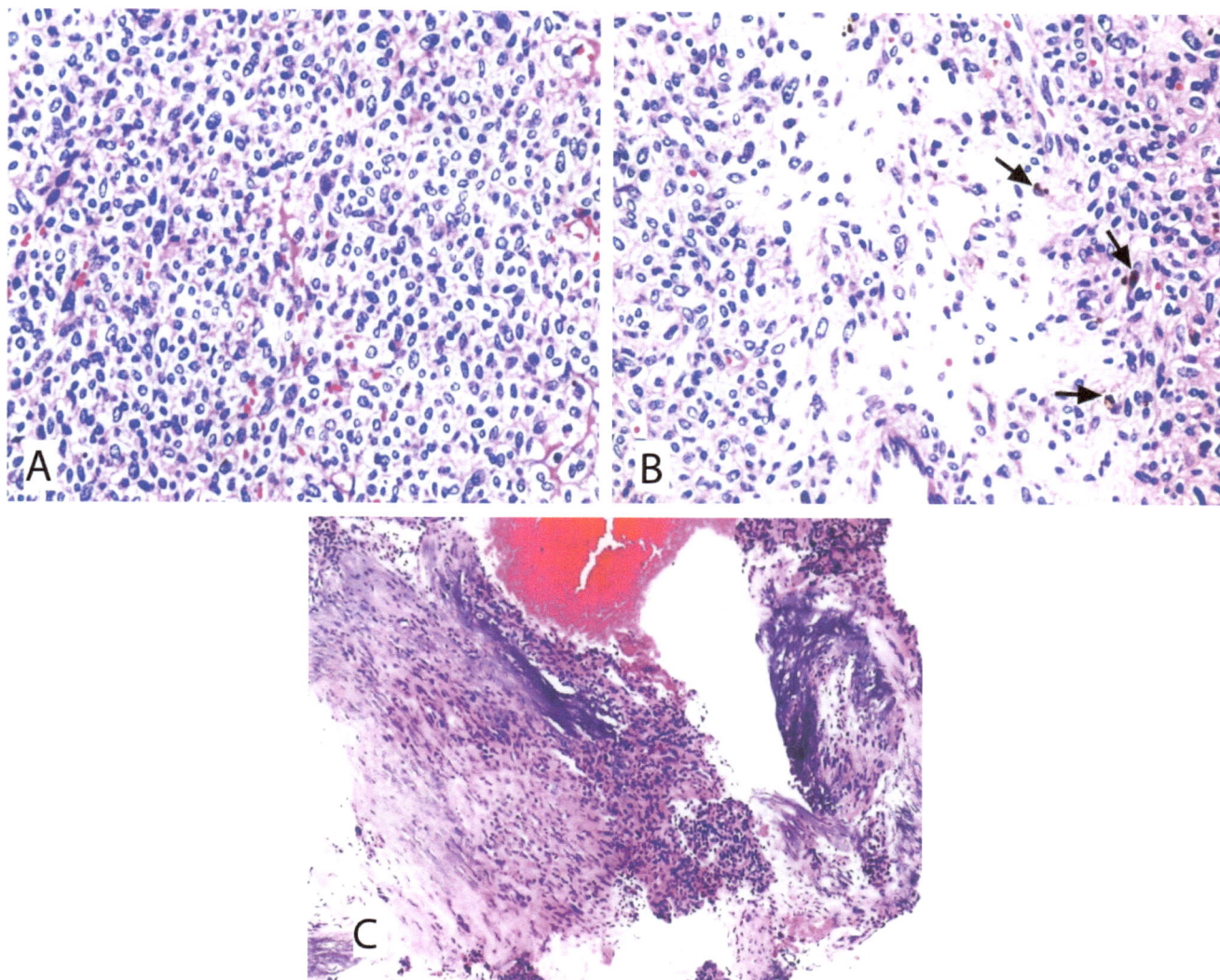

Fig. 10.7 A) sheets of bland tumor cells with rich capillary vasculature; (B) bland spindle cells with small nuclei lacking atypia or mitoses, note two siderophages (arrows) and (C) the typical 'grungy' calcified matrix.

It is now known that these PMT-MCT over express fibroblast growth factor-23 (FGP-23) which suppresses phosphate reabsorption by renal proximal tubular epithelial cells resulting in phosphaturia, hypophosphatemia and osteomalacia. FGP-23 can be demonstrated both by immunohistochemistry and RT-PCR[18]. Histological recognition of these tumors is important because most of these are benign tumors, their removal results in reversal of osteomalacia. Radiological features include severe osteomalacia and so-called pseudofractures (Fig. 10.8 A, B, C). Complete excision of the tumor and treatment for osteomalacia leads to healing of pseudofractures following phosphorous treatment. (Fig. 10.9)

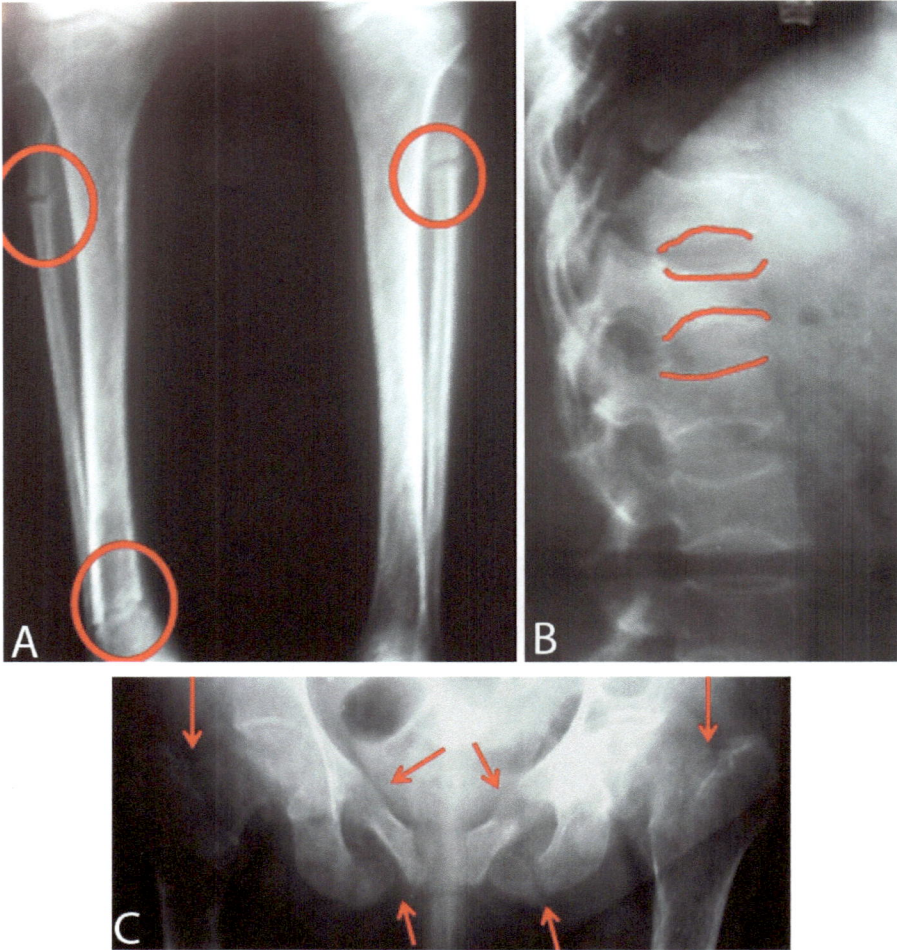

Fig 10.8 Pseudofractures A) x ray of both tibia and fibula shows diffuse osteopenia with pseudofractures: loser's zone in the proximal shaft of both fibula and distal shaft of right tibia B) X-ray of dorsal spine showing diffuse osteopenia with cod fish vertebrae. C) X ray of both hip joints showing diffuse osteopenia with multiple pseudofractures: losers zone in neck of both femora and superior as well as inferior pubic rami.

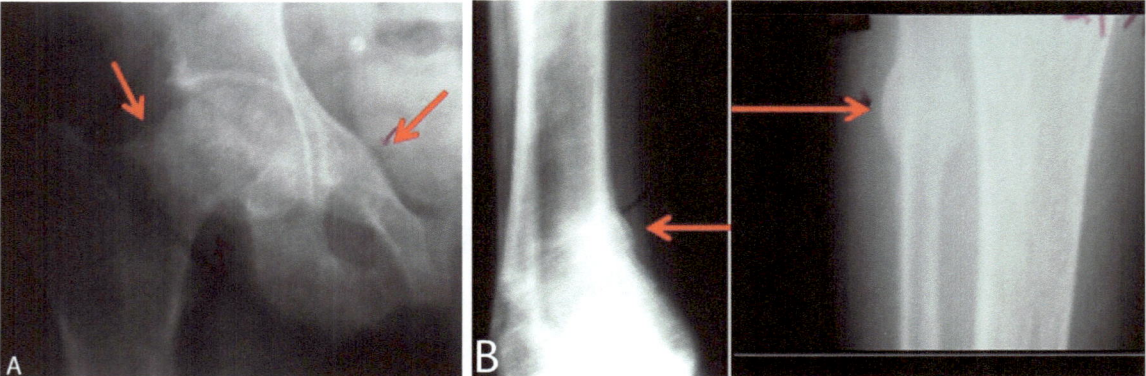

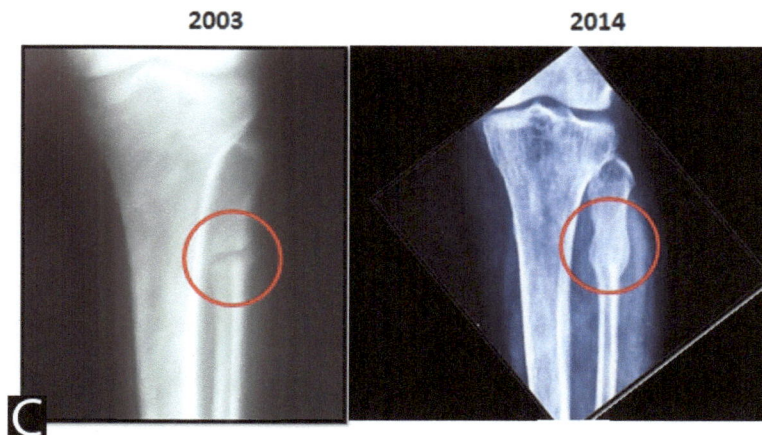

Fig 10.9 This illustration shows healing of pseudofractures following phosphorous treatment

References for Chapter 10

Giant cell reparative granuloma

1. Ratner V, Dorfman HD Giant cell reparative granuloma of the hand and foot bones Clin Orthop Relate Res 1990; 260:251-258

2. Jamil OA, Lechpammar mina, Prasad S, et al. Giant cell reparative granuloma of the sphenoid: Case report and review of the literature Surg neuro Int 2012; 3;140

3. Boedeker CC, Kayser G, Ridder GJ, et al Giant cell reparative granuloma of the temporal bone: A case report and review of literature Ear Nose Throat J; 2003:926-929

4. Ostrowasky ML, Spjut HJ. Lesions of bones of hands and feet Am J Surg Pathol 1997; 21:676-690

5. Yamaguchi T, Dorfinan HD. Giant cell reparative granuloma: A comparative clinicopathologic lesions in gnathic and extra gnathic sites Int j Surg Pathol 2001; 9;189-200

Aneurysmal bone cyst

6. Vergel De Dios AM, Bond JR, Shives T, et al. Aneurysmal Bone Cyst A Clinicopathologic Study of 238 Cases Cancer 1992; 69:2921-2931

7. Hudson TM Fluid levels in aneurysmal bone cysts: a CT feature AJM Am J Roentgenol 1984; 142:1001-1004

8. Levy WM, Miller AS, Bonakdarpour A, et al. Aneurysmal bone cyst secondary to other osseous lesions. Report of 57 cases Am J Clin Pathol 1975; 63:1-8

9. Martinez V, Sissons HA. Aneurysmal bone cyst A review of 123 cases including primary lesions and those secondary to other bone pathology Cancer 1988; 61:2291-2304

10. Sanerkin NG, Mott MG Roylance J. An unusual intraosseous lesion with fibroblastic, osteoclastic, osteoblastic, aneurysmal and fibromyxoid elements Cancer 1983; 52:2276-2286

11. Bertoni F, Bacchini P, Capanna R, et al. Solid variant of aneurysmal bone cyst Cancer 1993; 71:729-734

12. Savardekar AR, Patra D, Chatterjee D, et al Solid variant of aneurysmal bone cyst presenting as a giant cervical mass: A clinical, radiological, histopathological dilemma Surg Neurol Int. 2015; 6(Suppl 4): S182–S185.

Hyperparathyroidism/Brown tumor

13. Goswami P, Sarma P K, Sethi S, Hazarika S. Extensive skeletal manifestations in a case of primary hyperparathyroidism. Indian J Radiol Imaging 2002; 12:267-70
14. Francisco Bandeira1, Natalie E. Cusano2, Barbara C. Silva3, et al. Bone disease in primary hyperparathyroidism Arq Bras Endocrinol Metabolic. 2014; 58: 553–561.

Paget's disease of bone

15. Altman, R.D. Epidemiology of Paget's disease of bone. Clin Rev Bone Miner Metal 2002; 1: 99-102.
16. Ooi CG, Fraser WD. Paget's disease of bone Postgrad Med J. 1997; 73: 69–74

Phosphaturic mesenchymal tumor

17. Folpe AL, Fanburg-Smith J C, Billings' S D et al. Most osteomalacia-associated mesenchymal tumors are a single histopathologic entity: an analysis of 32 cases and a comprehensive review of the literature. Am J Surg Pathol. 2004; 28:1-30.
18. Armita B, Weiss, S W, Montogomery, E, et al. RT-PCR analysis for FGP -23 using paraffin sections to diagnose phosphaturic mesenchymal tumors with and without known tumor induced osteomalacia. Am J Surg Pathol 2009. 33:1348-1354.

Chapter 11: Molecular genetics of bone tumors

As in any other organ system, an accurate diagnosis of bone tumors is essential to predict biologic behavior, outcome and therefore therapeutic planning. Traditionally most pathologists find bone tumors difficult to diagnose for several reasons: bone tumors are rare, often have overlapping morphology, reactive / remodelling changes due to secondary fracture obscure underlying pathology, there is a need for radiological correlation, and the role of immunohistochemistry has been limited. These obstacles make conventional morphology the major basis of the diagnosis.

Over the past decade, understanding of molecular underpinnings of bone tumors has evolved considerably. Based on the current knowledge on recurrent molecular alterations of bone tumors, these can be globally grouped in three major types, namely, tumors with specific translocations combined with a relatively simple karyotype involving chromosomal translocations (Table 11.1), tumors with specific gene mutations or amplifications (Table 11.2, 11.3), and sarcomas with genetic instability and complex karyotypes (Table 11.4). There are some overlaps between these groups and not strictly separated based on above categories, e.g. secondary genetic alterations in TP53 or CDKN2A/B are observed in tumors with specific translocations.

Until recently, translocations were thought to be unique mechanisms of tumorigenesis in many sarcomas, hematolymphoid malignancies. With enhanced high thru put capabilities of genomic sequencing using next generation sequencing, RNA sequencing have uncovered many recurrent translocations and point mutations.

Different techniques are used for detecting genetic alterations depending on type of screening. For genomewide screening, conventional karyotyping, array comparative genomic hybridization and now whole exome / RNA sequencing using next generation sequencing (NGS) approach are commonly used. While targeted translocation detection is usually achieved by using fluorescent in-situ hybridization (FISH), reverse transcriptase polymerase chain reaction (RT-PCR) and NGS panels. In addition to diagnostic implications, the clinical importance includes potential targeted therapy.

Table 11.1: Balanced specific structural chromosomal translocations and gene fusions

Ewing sarcoma/PNET [1-6]	
t(11;22)(q24;q12)	EWSR1-FLI1 (85-95%)
t(21;22)(q22;q12)	EWSR1-ERG (5-15%)
t(7;22)(p22;q12)	EWSR1-ETV1 (<1%)
t(17;22)(q12;q12)	EWSR1-ETV4 (<1%)
t(2;22)(q33;q12)	EWSR1-FEV (<1%)
t(16;21)(p11;q22)	EWSR1-ERG (<1%)
t(2;16)(q35;p11)	EWSR1-FEV (<1%)

Table 11.1: Balanced specific structural chromosomal translocations and gene fusions continued.

Ewing sarcoma-like tumors / undifferentiated small round cell sarcomas	
t(6;22)(p21;q12)	EWSR1-POU5F1
inv(22)(q12)	EWSR1-ZSG (ZNF278)
t(4;22)(q31;q12)	EWSR1-SMARCA
t(2;22)(q31;q12)	EWSR1-SP3
t(1;22)(p36.1;q12)	EWS-ZNF278
t(4:19)(q35;q13.1), t(10;19)(q26.3;q13)	CIC/DUX4,
Recurrent paracentric inversion on chromosome X	BCOR/CCNB3
t(X;19)(q13;q13.3)	CIC/FOX04
Complex ring chromosome with amplification of the translocated segments	EWSR1-NFATc2
Aneurysmal bone cyst [7-13]	
t(16;17)(q22;p13)	CDH11-USP6 (Tre2)
t(1;17)(p34.1e34.3;p13)	TRAP150-USP6
t(3;17)(q21;p13)	ZNF9-USP6
t(9;17)(q22;p13)	OMD-USP6
t(17;17)(q12;p13)	COL1A1-USP6
Bizarre parosteal osteochondromatous proliferation (Nora lesion) [14]	
t(1;17)(q32;q21)	RDC1
Epithelioid hemangioendothelioma [15-17]	
t(1;3)(p36;q25)	WWTR1-CAMTA1
Mesenchymal chondrosarcoma [24]	
Del(8)(q13q21)	HEY1-NCOA2
Myoepithelial tumor of bone [25-26]	
t(6;22)(p21;q12)	EWSR1-POU5F1
t(19;22)(q13;q12)	EWSR1-ZNF444
t(1;22)(q23;q12)	EWSR1-PBX1
Subungual exostosis [27]	
t(X;6)(q24-q26;q15-21)	COL12A1-COL4A5

Table 11.2: Specific amplifications/gains

Low grade (parosteal and intramedullary) osteosarcoma [41-47]	
12q14-15 (ring/marker chromosome)	CDK4, MDM2, HMGA2, GLI, SAS
Chordoma [39,40]	
6q27	T

Table 11.3 Specific gene mutations

Enchondroma, central and periosteal chondrosarcoma [34-38]	IDH1, IDH2
Fibrous dysplasia [18-23]	GNAS
Osteochondroma [28-33]	EXT1, EXT2

Table 11.4: Tumors with complex karyotype and mutations

Osteosarcoma [41-47]	Extremely genetically unstable with complex amplifications, translocations, deletions TP53, RB, MDM2, CHK2
Ewing sarcoma-like tumors	Complex ring chromosome with amplification of the translocated segments

References for Chapter 11: Molecular genetic pathology of Bone tumors

Ewing's sarcoma / PNET

1. Sankar S, Lessnick SL. Promiscuous partnerships in Ewing's sarcoma. Cancer Genet 2011;204:351e365
2. Savola S, Nardi F, Scotlandi K, et al. Microdeletions in 9p21.3 induce false negative results in CDKN2A FISH analysis of Ewing sarcoma. Cytogenet Genome Res 2007;119:21e26.
3. Graham C, Chilton-MacNeill S, Zielenska M, et al. The CIC-DUX4 fusion transcript is present in a subgroup of pediatric primitive round cell sarcomas. Hum Pathol 2012; 43:180e189.
4. Italiano A, Sung YS, Zhang L, et al. High prevalence of CIC fusion with double-homeobox (DUX4) transcription factors in EWSR1-negative undifferentiated small blue round cell sarcomas. Genes Chromosomes Cancer 2012; 51:207e218.
5. Szuhai K, Ijszenga M, de Jong D, et al. The NFATc2 gene is involved in a novel cloned translocation in a Ewing sarcoma variant that couples its function in immunology to oncology. Clin Cancer Res 2009; 15:2259e2268.
6. Machado I, Navarro L, Pellin A, Navarro S, Agaimy A, Tardío JC, Karseladze A, Petrov S, Scotlandi K, Picci P, Llombart-Bosch A. Defining Ewing and Ewing-like small round cell tumors (SRCT): The need for molecular techniques in their categorization and differential diagnosis. A study of 200 cases. Ann Diagn Pathol. 2016 Jun;22:25-32. doi: 0.1016/j.anndiagpath.2016.03.002. Epub 2016 Mar 14. PubMed PMID: 27180056.

Aneurysmal bone cysts

7. Panoutsakopoulos G, Pandis N, Kyriazoglou I, et al. Recurrent t(16;17)(q22;p13) in aneurysmal bone cysts. Genes Chromosomes Cancer 1999; 26:265e266. Oliveira AM, Hsi BL, Weremowicz S, et al. USP6 (Tre2) fusion oncogenes in aneurysmal bone cyst. Cancer Res 2004;64: 1920e1923.
8. Oliveira AM, Perez-Atayde AR, Dal Cin P, et al. Aneurysmal bone cyst variant translocations upregulate USP6 transcription by promoter swapping with the ZNF9, COL1A1, TRAP150, and OMD genes. Oncogene 2005; 24:3419e3426.
9. Ye Y, Pringle LM, Lau AW, et al. TRE17/USP6 oncogene translocated in aneurysmal bone cyst induces matrix metalloproteinase production via activation of NF-kappaB. Oncogene 2010; 29:3619e3629.
10. Lau AW, Pringle LM, Quick L, et al. TRE17/ubiquitin-specific protease 6 (USP6) oncogene translocated in aneurysmal bone cyst blocks osteoblastic maturation via an autocrine mechanism involving bone morphogenetic protein dysregulation. J Biol Chem 2010 Nov 19;285(47):37111e37120.

11. Oliveira AM, Perez-Atayde AR, Inwards CY, et al. USP6 and CDH11 oncogenes identify the neoplastic cell in primary aneurysmal bone cysts and are absent in so-called secondary aneurysmal bone cysts. Am J Pathol 2004; 165:1773e1780.
12. Sukov WR, Franco MF, Erickson-Johnson M, et al. Frequency of USP6 rearrangements in myositis ossificans, brown tumor, and cherubism: molecular cytogenetic evidence that a subset of "myositis ossificans-like lesions" are the early phases in the formation of soft-tissue aneurysmal bone cyst. Skeletal Radiol 2008; 37:321e327.
13. Erickson-Johnson MR, Chou MM, Evers BR, et al. Nodular fasciitis: a novel model of transient neoplasia induced by MYH9-USP6 gene fusion. Lab Invest 2011; 91:1427e1433.

Bizarre parosteal osteochondromatous proliferation (Nora lesion):

14. Kuruvilla S, Marco R, Raymond AK, Al-Ibraheemi A, Tatevian N. Bizarre Parosteal Osteochondromatous Proliferation (Nora's lesion) with translocation t(1;17)(q32;q21): a case report and role of cytogenetic studies on diagnosis. Ann Clin Lab Sci. 2011 Summer;41(3):285-7. PubMed PMID: 22075515.

Epithelioid hemangioendothelioma

15. Errani C, Zhang L, Sung YS, et al. A novel WWTR1-CAMTA1 gene fusion is a consistent abnormality in epithelioid hemangioendothelioma of different anatomic sites. Genes Chromosomes Cancer 2011; 50:644e653.
16. Mendlick MR, Nelson M, Pickering D, et al. Translocation t(1; 3)(p36.3;q25) is a nonrandom aberration in epithelioid hemangioendothelioma. Am J Surg Pathol 2001; 25:684e687.
17. Tanas MR, Sboner A, Oliveira AM, et al. Identification of a disease-defining gene fusion in epithelioid hemangioendothelioma. Sci Transl Med 2011; 3:98.

Fibrous dysplasia:

18. Dal Cin P, Sciot R, Brys P, et al. Recurrent chromosome aberrations in fibrous dysplasia of the bone: a report of the CHAMP study group. Chromosomes and Morphology. Cancer Genet Cytogenet 2000;122:30e32.
19. Idowu BD, Al-Adnani M, O'Donnell P, et al. A sensitive mutation specific screening technique for GNAS1 mutations in cases of fibrous dysplasia: the first report of a codon 227 mutation in bone. Histopathology 2007;50:691e704.
20. Delaney D, Diss TC, Presneau N, et al. GNAS1 mutations occur more commonly than previously thought in intramuscular myxoma. Mod Pathol 2009; 22:718e724.
21. Pollandt K, Engels C, Kaiser E, et al. Gsalpha gene mutations in monostotic fibrous dysplasia of bone and fibrous dysplasia-like low-grade central osteosarcoma. Virchows Arch 2001;439: 170e175.
22. Sakamoto A, Oda Y, Iwamoto Y, et al. A comparative study of fibrous dysplasia and osteofibrous dysplasia with regard to Gsalpha mutation at the Arg201 codon: polymerase chain reaction-restriction fragment length polymorphism analysis of paraffin-embedded tissues. J Mol Diagn 2000; 2:67e72.
23. Toyosawa S, Yuki M, Kishino M, Ogawa Y, et al. Ossifying fibroma vs fibrous dysplasia of the jaw: molecular and immunological characterization. Mod Pathol 2007; 20:389e396.

Mesenchymal chondrosarcoma

24. WangL, Motoi T, Khanin R, et al. Identification of a novel, recurrentHEY1-NCOA2 fusion in mesenchymal chondrosarcoma based ona genome-wide screen of exon-level expression data. Genes Chromosomes Cancer 2012;51:127e139.

Myoepithelial tumor of bone

25. Antonescu CR, Zhang L, Chang NE, Pawel BR, Travis W, Katabi N, Edelman M,Rosenberg AE, Nielsen GP, Dal Cin P, Fletcher CD. EWSR1-POU5F1 fusion in soft tissue myoepithelial tumors. A molecular analysis of sixty-six cases, including soft tissue, bone, and visceral lesions, showing common involvement of the EWSR1 gene. Genes Chromosomes Cancer. 2010 Dec;49(12):1114-24. doi: 10.1002/gcc.20819.
26. PubMed PMID: 20815032; PubMed Central PMCID: PMC3540416.

Subungual exostosis

27. Storlazzi CT, Wozniak A, Panagopoulos I, Sciot R, Mandahl N, Mertens F, Debiec-Rychter M. Rearrangement of the COL12A1 and COL4A5 genes in subungual exostosis: molecular cytogenetic delineation of the tumor-specific translocation t(X;6) (q13-14;q22). Int J Cancer. 2006 Apr 15;118(8):1972-6. PubMed PMID: 16284948.

Osteochondromas (Exostosis)

28. Ahn J, Ludecke H-J, Lindow S, et al. Cloning of the putative tumor suppressor gene for hereditary multiple exostoses (EXT1). Nature Genet 1995; 11:137e143.
29. Stickens D, Clines G, Burbee D, et al. The EXT2 multiple exostoses gene defines a family of putative tumor suppressor genes. Nature Genet 1996; 14:25e32.
30. Bovee JVMG, Cleton-Jansen AM, Wuyts W, et al. EXT-mutation analysis and loss of heterozygosity in sporadic and hereditary osteochondromas and secondary chondrosarcomas. Am J Hum Genet 1999;65:689e698.
31. Hameetman L, Szuhai K, Yavas A, et al. The role of EXT1 in non-hereditary osteochondroma: identification of homozygous deletions. J Natl Cancer Inst 2007; 99:396e406.
32. Szuhai K, Jennes I, de Jong D, et al. Tiling resolution array-CGH shows that somatic mosaic deletion of the EXT gene is causative in EXT gene mutation negative multiple osteochondromas patients. Hum Mutat 2011; 32:2036e2049.
33. Jennes I, de Jong D, Mees K, et al. Breakpoint characterization of large deletions in EXT1 or EXT2 in 10 Multiple Osteochondromas families. BMC Med Genet 2011; 12:85.

Enchondroma, central chondrosarcoma and central and periosteal chondromas:

34. Amary MF, Bacsi K, Maggiani F, et al. IDH1 and IDH2 mutations are frequent events in central chondrosarcoma and central and periosteal chondromas but not in other mesenchymal tumors. J Pathol 2011; 224:334e343.
35. Pansuriya TC, van Eijk R, d'Adamo P, et al. Somatic mosaic IDH1 and IDH2 mutations are associated with enchondroma and spindle cell hemangioma in Ollier disease and Maffucci syndrome. Nat Genet 2011; 43:1256e1261.
36. Amary MF, Damato S, Halai D, et al. Ollier disease and Maffucci syndrome are caused by somatic mosaic mutations of IDH1 and IDH2. Nat Genet 2011; 43:1262e1265.
37. Arai M, Nobusawa S, Ikota H, Takemura S, Nakazato Y. Frequent IDH1/2 mutations in intracranial chondrosarcoma: a possible diagnostic clue for its differentiation from chordoma. Brain Tumor Pathol 2012
38. Damato S, Alorjani M, Bonar F, et al. IDH1 mutations are not found in cartilaginous tumors other than central and periosteal chondrosarcomas and enchondromas. Histopathology 2012;60: 363e365.

Chordoma:

39. Yang XR, Ng D, Alcorta DA, et al. T (brachyury) gene duplication confers major susceptibility to familial chordoma. Nat Genet 2009; 41:1176e1178.
40. Presneau N, Shalaby A, Ye H, et al. Role of the transcription factor T (brachyury) in the pathogenesis of sporadic chordoma: a genetic and functional-based study. J Pathol 2011; 223:327e335.

Osteosarcoma:

41. Stock C, Kager L, Fink FM, et al. Chromosomal regions involved in the pathogenesis of osteosarcomas. Genes Chromosomes Cancer 2000; 28:329e336.
42. Selvarajah S, Yoshimoto M, Ludkovski O, et al. Genomic signatures of chromosomal instability and osteosarcoma progression detected by high resolution array CGH and interphase FISH. Cytogenet Genome Res 2008; 122:5e15.
43. Wunder JS, Gokgoz N, Parkes R, et al. TP53 mutations and outcome in osteosarcoma: a prospective, multicenter study. J Clin Oncol 2005; 23:1483e1490.
44. Miller CW, Ikezoe T, Krug U, et al. Mutations of the CHK2gene are found in some osteosarcomas, but are rare in breast, lung, and ovarian tumors. Genes Chromosomes Cancer 2002; 33:17e21.
45. Mohseny AB, Szuhai K, Romeo S, et al. Osteosarcoma originates from mesenchymal stem cells in consequence of aneuploidization and genomic loss of Cdkn2. J Pathol 2009; 219: 294e305.
46. Ulaner GA, Huang HY, Otero J, et al. Absence of a telomere maintenance mechanism as a favorable prognostic factor in patients with osteosarcoma. Cancer Res 2003; 63:1759e1763. 97. Sanders RP, Drissi R, Billups CA, et al. Telomerase expression predicts unfavorable outcome in osteosarcoma. J Clin Oncol 2004; 22:3790e3797.
47. Mohseny AB, Tieken C, Van der Velden PA, et al. Small deletions but not methylation underlie CDKN2A/p16 loss of expression in conventional osteosarcoma. Genes Chromosomes Cancer 2010; 49:1095e1103.
